KT-415-977

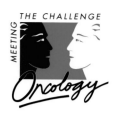

THE CHALLENGE
MEETING
Oncology

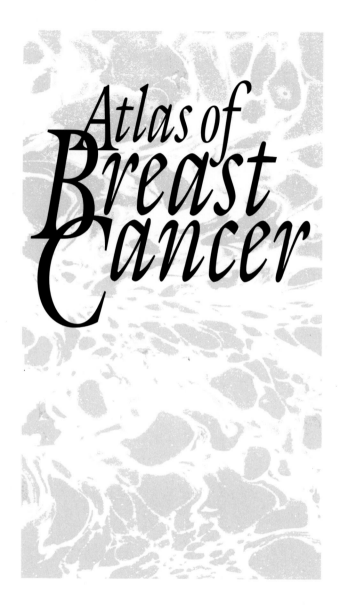

Atlas of Breast Cancer

Presented with the compliments of

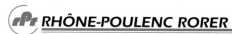 RHÔNE-POULENC RORER

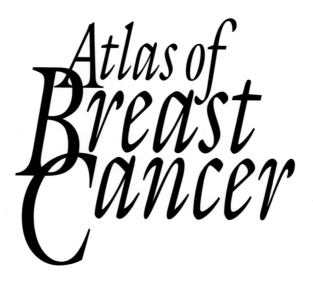

Atlas of Breast Cancer

editor

Daniel F. Hayes, MD

Medical Director
Breast Evaluation Center
Dana–Farber Cancer Institute
Assistant Professor of Medicine
Harvard Medical School
Boston, Massachusetts

foreword by

I. Craig Henderson, MD

Professor of Medicine
Chief, Medical Oncology
Director, Clinical Oncology Programs
UCSF Cancer Center, Mt. Zion
University of California, San Francisco
San Francisco, California

Mosby-Wolfe

London Baltimore Bogotá Boston Buenos Aires Caracas Carlsbad, CA Chicago Madrid Mexico City Milan Naples, FL New York Philadelphia St. Louis Sydney Tokyo Toronto Wiesbaden

Published in 1993 by
Mosby—Year Book Europe Limited.
Reprinted 1995 by Mosby—Wolfe,
an imprint of Times Mirror International Publishers Ltd.

For full details of all Times Mirror International Publishers Limited please write to
Times Mirror International Publishers Limited, 7–12 Tavistock Square,
London, WC1H 9LB, England.

Library of Congresss Cataloging-in-Publication Data
Atlas of breast cancer / editor, Daniel F. Hayes.
p. cm.
Includes bibliographical references and index.
ISBN 1-56375-010-4
1. Breast—Cancer—Atlases. I. Hayes, Daniel, 1951–
[DNLM: 1. Breast Neoplasms—atlases. WP 17 A8785]
RC280.B8A85 1993
616.99'449—dc20
92–49328

British Library Cataloging-in-Publication Data
A catalogue record for this book is available from the British Library.

Editor/Project Manager: Leah Kennedy
Editorial Assistant: David Yoon
Art Director: Kathryn Armstrong
Designers: Selina Bank, Jennifer Bergamini
Illustration Director: Laura Pardi Duprey
Illustrator: Sue Ann Fung-Ho

Printed in Hong Kong by Everbest Printing Company, Inc.

10 9 8 7 6 5 4 3 2

To George P. Canellos, MD, who first stimulated my interest in breast cancer; and to I. Craig Henderson, MD, who immersed me in the pool of clinical, scientific, and educational aspects of breast cancer, and who was the stimulus for many of the concepts in this book.

Acknowledgments

Many of the photomicrographs used in this atlas were initially published in *Atlas of Diagnostic Oncology*, edited by Dr. Arthur Skarin. These photomicrographs were supplied by Dr. Robert Penney, Associate Pathologist, The Community Hospital of Indianapolis in Indiana. Much gratitude goes to Dr. William Kaplan, Chief of Nuclear Medicine, who supplied expertise, cases, and radionuclide scans throughout the text.

I would also like to acknowledge Ms. Leah Kennedy, the editor for this project, whose patience and prodding have been instrumental in the publication of this text. In addition, I would like to thank Ms. Sue Ann Fung-Ho, the medical illustrator, who was able to convert many of my haphazard concepts into understandable illustrations. Finally, I would like to thank Ms. Teri Guidi, who has kept my life organized during the preparation of the atlas.

Preface

As an academician, I am frequently called upon to discuss the diagnosis and treatment of breast cancer with my patients, students, and colleagues. Whether these discussions are held in the context of formal teaching lectures or impromptu hallway consults, I find myself relying heavily on a variety of "props," most often consisting of photographic slides or hastily scribbled diagrams, tables, and figures scrawled on the nearest chalkboard and/or available piece of paper (not uncommonly the back of a divider in a patient's medical record). These interactions have made it obvious that conveyence of information involving breast cancer is clearly a visual process.

The *Atlas of Breast Cancer* is a compilation of concepts gathered by my-self and my colleagues in the Breast Evaluation Center at the Dana Farber Cancer Institute and surrounding institutions over the last several years, illustrated by specific cases. We have attempted to address established clinical standards as well as controversial issues that cover the gamut of caring for women who are at risk for or who actually have breast cancer. Although the authors frequently cite published literature to discuss certain situations, comprehensive reviews of each issue are beyond the design of this atlas. Indeed, so the reader can further investigate the topic, suggested readings are included after each chapter. More detailed sources, to which frequent references are made, include *Breast Diseases*, edited by Harris, Hellman, Henderson, and Kinne, and *Cancer: Principles and Practice of Oncology*, by DeVita, Hellman, and Rosenberg.

The focus of the atlas is to introduce the student or non-oncologist physician to the important features and concepts of each aspect of breast cancer. The oncologist may also find this volume useful, most likely to illustrate a salient point while discussing etiology, screening and diagnosis, primary and adjuvant treatment, and evaluation and treatment of metastatic disease in patients with breast cancer.

The fields of breast cancer research are moving rapidly. New diagnostic tests are being developed to detect genetic propensies for the disease, and improved imaging technologies for screening are on the horizon. With the demonstration that breast-preserving approaches are as effective and appropriate as mastectomy, efforts are ongoing to improve cosmetic outcomes. We have now advanced past the initial controversy generated around the success of adjuvant systemic therapy, and large clinical investigations are now aimed at "fine-tuning" patient selection and specific therapies. Moreover, recent advances in molecular biology and in the understanding of the physiology of breast cancer promise even more effective and less toxic therapies than are currently available. All in all, we are in the midst of an exciting era of breast cancer research that should lead to substantial benefits for our patients. In order to exploit these advances, a fundamental knowledge of the basic and clinical aspects of the disease is essential for all health care providers. It is hoped that the atlas will, in part, provide the platform on which to build such a fund of knowledge.

Daniel F. Hayes, MD

Foreword

Although breast cancer is the most frequently encountered cancer in women and is second only to lung cancer as a source of cancer mortality in women, a mere recitation of the incidence figures belied the importance of this disease to practicing physicians of all specialties. It is estimated that more than 180,000 women will be diagnosed with breast cancer in 1992. However, somewhere between 900,000 and 1.8 million American women will undergo a breast biopsy. The number of women who will present to physicians with concern either because of a lump in the breast or because of a perception that they are at high risk of developing breast cancer cannot be accurately ascertained, but it is plausible that it is at least ten times the number of women who actually undergo biopsy. Thus, it is reasonable to assume that 10 to 20 million women in the United States will seek the consultations of a physician for some problem related to the breast in 1992.

Breast cancer is characterized by a long history and marked heterogeneity in growth rates and clinical manifestations. It is estimated that the preclinical course of breast cancer is between five and ten years for most patients and that the interval from the point when the cancer can be diagnosed by mammography but not by physical examination or symptoms to the time when the cancer is 1 cm in diameter is in a range of several years for most patients. The clinical course ranges from five to 40 years, and it is not unusual for patients to recur more than five years after the initial diagnosis. During the course of the disease most patients will receive treatment from a surgeon, a radiotherapist, and a medical oncologist. In addition, they usually require the expertise of pathologists, plastic surgeons, nurse specialists, and social workers. In this context, it is not surprising that the number of studies reported each year appears to be growing at a rate that may actually exceed the growth of the breast cancer epidemic itself.

Few, if any, other diseases have been studied so carefully with randomized trials. In fact, two of the first randomized trials evaluated adjuvant radiotherapy and adjuvant ovarian ablation following mastectomy and were initiated in 1948 at the dawn of the modern era, during which the randomized clinical trial has become a gold standard. In adjuvant systemic treatment studies alone, more than 80,000 women have been radomized in approximately 100 separate trials published on one or more occasions. A similar number of studies are ongoing or as yet unpublished. Making sense of this information is a full-time occupation for dedicated group specialists and a difficult challenge for those who do not devote their entire effort to the treatment of breast cancer. For this reason, books such as this atlas are an important part of the medical literature of breast cancer.

In the chapters that follow, Dr. Hayes and his colleagues provide a succinct, readily accessible, and cohesive summary of the state of the art, with particular emphasis on a graphic presentation of the fundamental principles of diagnosis and treatment. It is not merely a collection of essays on breast cancer, since these physicians have worked closely together in a team effort as part of the Breast Evaluation Center at the Dana–Farber Cancer Institute in Boston. As a consequence, information is presented with a shared underlying philosophy and approach to the disease. However, because of the reliance on objective observations made from randomized trials addressing the appropriate primary treatment, adjuvant therapy, and selection of palliative approaches to the patient with a systemic metastases, the information can be accepted as more than just an opinion of recognized experts but a true statement of our current knowledge about this complex disease.

I. Craig Henderson, MD

Contents

Contributors

T.J. Eberlein, MD
Chief, Division of Surgical Oncology
Director, Biologic Cancer Therapy Program
Brigham and Women's Hospital
Surgical Director
Breast Evaluation Center
Dana–Farber Cancer Institute
Associate Professor of Surgery
Harvard Medical School
Boston, Massachusetts

Daniel F. Hayes, MD
Medical Director
Breast Evaluation Center
Dana–Farber Cancer Institute
Assistant Professor of Medicine
Harvard Medical School
Boston, Massachusetts

Abram Recht, MD
Associate Professor
Joint Center for Radiotherapy
Department of Radiation Oncology
Harvard Medical School
Boston, Massachusetts

Stuart J. Schnitt, MD
Associate Director of Surgical Pathology
Beth Israel Hospital
Consultant in Pathology
Dana–Farber Cancer Institute
Assistant Professor of Pathology
Harvard Medical School
Boston, Massachusetts

Paul C. Stomper, MD
Director of Diagnostic Radiology
Roswell Park Cancer Institute
Associate Professor in Radiology
School of Medicine and Biomedical Sciences
State University of New York at Buffalo
Buffalo, New York

Editor of Photographs
Arthur T. Skarin, MD
Medical Oncology Division
Associate Professor of Medicine
Harvard Medical School
Boston, Massachusetts

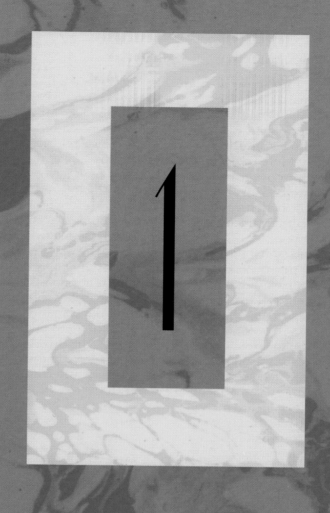

Introduction to Breast Cancer

Daniel F. Hayes

Breast cancer is an extraordinarily important disease in the Western world. Over 150,000 women are diagnosed each year in the United States alone, and roughly one-third of them will die of breast cancer. However, breast cancer affects not only the potential long-term survival rate of patients but also their cosmetic and emotional well-being. Moreover, the psychologic and physical consequences of breast cancer have a far-reaching social impact on relatives, friends, and associates in the home and in the workplace. Almost no one in our society is entirely unaffected by breast cancer.

Over the last 30 to 40 years, substantial progress has been made in the diagnosis and treatment of breast cancer. Furthermore, dramatic efforts have been made to detect "risk factors" that will help to identify those women likely to develop breast cancer and the genetic factors that contribute to these risks. These studies have led to investigations regarding the multiple causes of breast cancer and have generated efforts to prevent it.

This *Atlas* presents, in a graphic manner, the basic concepts of the causes, diagnosis, and treatment of breast cancer. The *Atlas* not only emphasizes the surgical and medical approaches devoted to these advances but also outlines the important contributions toward preservation or restoration of cosmetic integrity that are so important to the overall well-being of patients with this disease. Chapter 2 deals with the potential causes of breast cancer and the identification of women who are at higher risk. The discussion of normal breast development and anatomy in Chapter 3 leads into a description of both the techniques and the results of screening and diagnostic mammography (Chapter 4). Chapters 5 through 9 illustrate the importance of multimodality interactions in the diagnosis and treatment of breast cancer, with an emphasis on achieving an acceptable cosmetic outcome while preventing recurrence. Chapters 10 and 11 discuss advances over the last 20 years in the use of systemic therapy (both endocrine and chemotherapy). These chapters include the major successes that have been realized by the use of early adjuvant therapy to prevent relapse. Finally, in Chapter 12, local and systemic therapy for the treatment of recurrent (metastatic) disease is discussed in detail, in the context of the various diagnostic techniques used for detection of metastatic disease.

Breast cancer is an extremely heterogeneous disease. For example, the most clearly identified risk factors for its development are gender (female) and age (over 50 years). However, more than 75 percent of women with newly diagnosed breast cancer do not have any of the other known risk factors (such as a positive family history). This implies that the etiology of breast cancer is probably multifactorial, including both inherited and acquired factors. Although these interacting factors ultimately generate invasive malignancy, they almost certainly lead to a variety of genetic changes that produce variable biologic behaviors from one patient to the next. These differences produce a broad spectrum of clinical situations that makes sweeping, generalized statements about the behavior of breast cancer difficult, if not impossible. This heterogeneity is the source of much of the confusion and controversy that have surrounded the study and treatment of breast cancer over the years. The diverse characteristics of carcinoma of the breast have underscored the importance of designing concurrently controlled clinical trials in order to reach satisfactory treatment recommendations.

The study of breast cancer has been dominated by one of two schools of thought. During the first three quarters of this century, most physicians assumed that breast cancer began in the epithelium of the breast, remained localized for a period of time, and then spread in an orderly fashion to regional targets such as skin and lymph nodes, and finally to distant organs (Fig. 1.1). This concept, championed by Dr. Halsted, led to extremely aggressive local approaches to therapy, included the so-called "radical mastectomy" and/or the addition of postmastectomy radiation therapy.

Several clinical trials testing the Halsted theory demonstrated that although increasingly intense local therapy decreases the risk of local recurrence, it does not decrease the rate of distant recurrence or the overall rate of survival. These results led to a second theory that breast cancer may become metastatic very early in its course. According to this theory, most if not all patients with newly diagnosed primary breast cancers also have widespread, systemic micrometastases. Regional lymph node involvement serves as a marker, not a barrier, for distant metastases (Fig. 1.2). This theory led to the study of adjuvant systemic therapy (see Chapter 11).

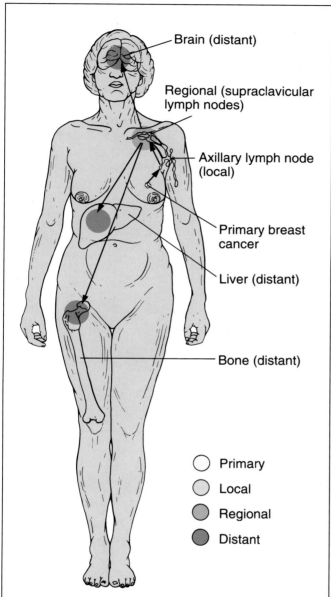

Figure 1.1 Halsted theory of breast cancer spread. This theory suggests that breast cancer originates in the breast, eventually spreads to local skin and/or lymph nodes, and then ultimately affects distant organs. This theory maintains that local/regional lymph nodes serve as "barriers" to the spread of metastatic breast cancer. The implication of this theory is that more intensive local therapy should lead to an increased rate of cures.

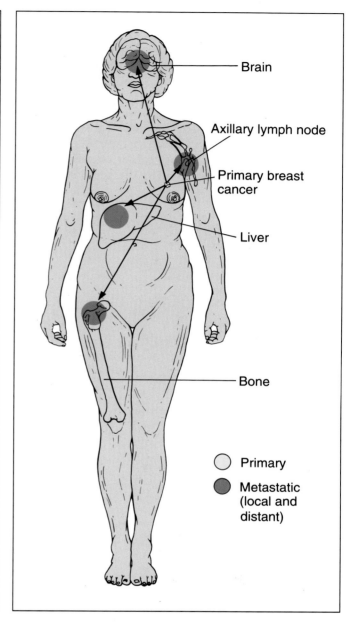

Figure 1.2 Systemic theory of breast cancer spread. This theory suggests that breast cancer becomes metastatic very early in its course, once invasion through the basement membrane of the duct or lobule has occurred. This theory maintains that local therapy will have few if any long-term effects on survival, since the disease is already systemic at the time of diagnosis.

Introduction to Breast Cancer

In reality, because of the heterogeneity of breast cancer, both of these theories are partially correct. For example, as reviewed in Chapter 4, several studies have suggested that screening mammography and local therapy alone result in improved survival for approximately 20 percent of patients. Thus, in certain patients breast cancer remains noninvasive or invasive but localized during a period of its natural history before becoming metastatic, and local therapy alone during this time is curative. In fact, a subset of patients may have disease that is confined to the regional lymph nodes without distant metastases. Nevertheless, many other patients are not cured by local therapy even with earlier diagnosis, and therefore they may benefit more from systemic therapy. These concepts are illustrated in Figure 1.3.

Even as we become more sophisticated in the technology of diagnostic studies, primary surgery, radiotherapy, and systemic therapy, it is still unclear which combination or combinations of modalities are optimal for the treatment of patients with breast cancer. It seems logical that those patients with disease still confined to

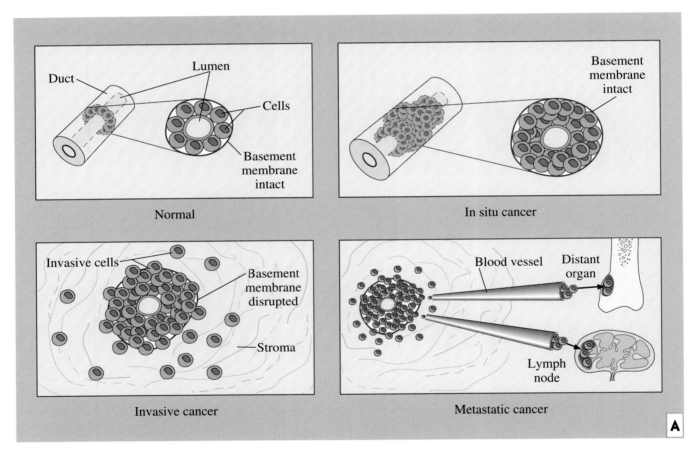

Figure 1.3 (A) Time line of breast cancer suggesting probable heterogeneity. Primary breast cancers begin as single (or more) cells which have lost normal regulation of differentiation and proliferation but remain confined within the basement membrane of the duct or lobule. As these cells go through several doublings, at some point they invade through the basement membrane of the ductule or lobule and ultimately metastasize to distant organs.

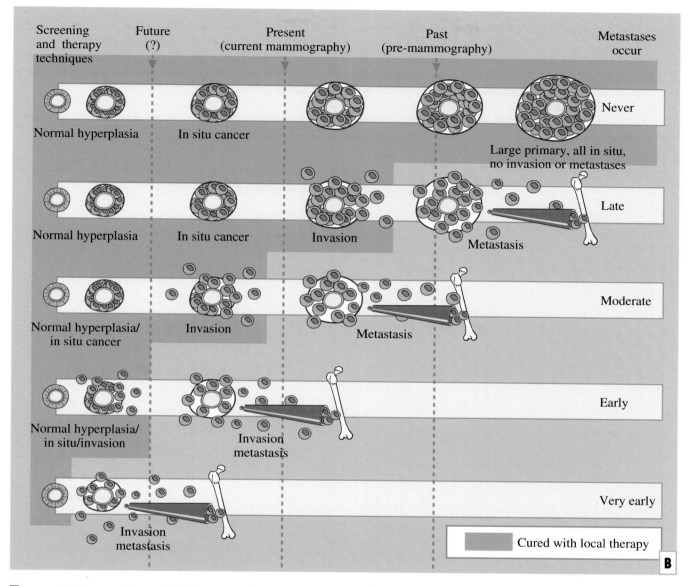

Figure 1.3, continued (B) These events may occur very early or very late, or at any time in between, during the development of the primary tumor, resulting in tremendous heterogeneity in the clinical presentation for individual patients. Therefore, some patients' disease remains localized until very late in their initial course, whereas other patients are destined to die of metastatic disease regardless of when their primary breast cancer is detected.

the breast should benefit principally from limited, locally applied therapy, whereas those with widespread systemic disease should benefit primarily from systemic therapies. It is those patients with minimally microscopic metastases who may stand to benefit most from a combination of both local and systemic therapy, especially if, as outlined in Chapter 10, systemic therapy is most effective before the development of grossly metastatic disease (Fig. 1.4).

It is not the intent of this *Atlas* to provide detailed descriptions of the various studies concerning breast cancer. In this regard, the reader is frequently referred to resources in which such details are presented. Rather, this *Atlas* is designed for the student, physician, and even the oncologist who wishes to have access to a more graphic depiction of the concepts of this disease and the various modalities that can be used to evaluate and treat it effectively.

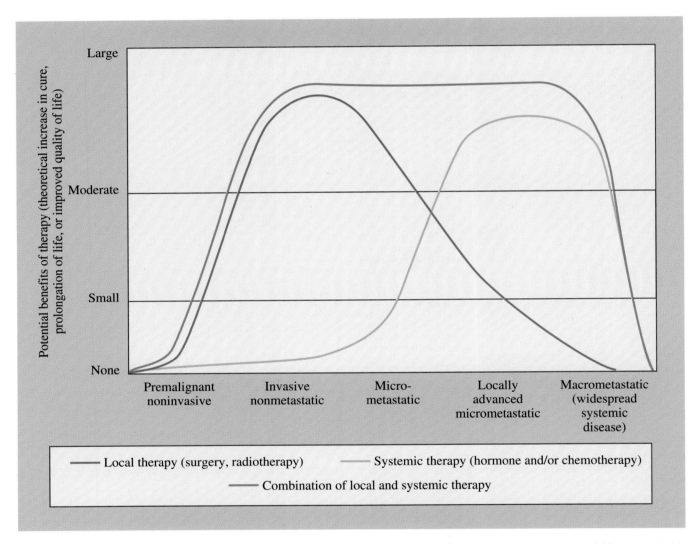

Figure 1.4 Potential benefits of local and/or systemic therapy depending on the patient's stage. Local therapy would be expected to be most effective at a time when the patient's disease is confined within the ducts or lobules (premalignant or noninvasive) or is only minimally invasive. Local therapy would be expected to have little if any effect in patients with widespread systemic disease (macrometastatic), except in specific cases of isolated organ sites requiring palliation. Systemic therapy would be expected to have its greatest effect in prolonging survival in patients who are most likely to have distant metastases but whose disease has not had an opportunity to develop substantial resistance (micrometastatic), which might develop with ongoing tumor growth.

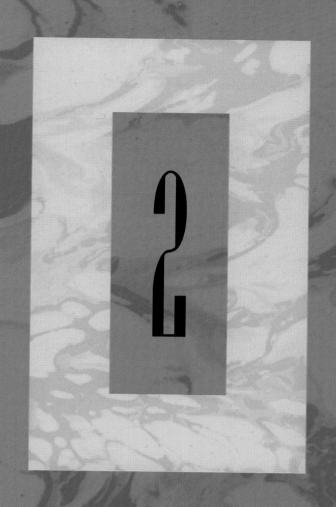

2

Risk Factors, Epidemiology, and Development of Breast Cancer

Daniel F. Hayes and Stuart J. Schnitt

There are at least two reasons to identify certain factors that predict which members of a population are at risk for a given disease. First, if treatment of the disease is more successful when applied early in the course rather than late, then monitoring efforts can be focused on those individuals most likely to develop the disease. Second, information about identifiable risk factors may provide insight into the pathogenesis of the disease, leading to more productive research and perhaps to improved prevention or treatment.

The two most important identifiable risk factors for breast cancer are gender and age. The incidence of breast cancer among women in the developed Western world is approximately 200 to 250 per 100,000 women per year. Moreover, the incidence of breast cancer in women increases with age (Fig. 2.1). Unfortunately, more than 70 percent of women over the age of 50 who present with breast cancer do not have any other identifiable risk factors. Therefore, although risk fac-

tors other than gender and age have been identified, they account for only a small percentage of patients with the disease. For this reason, an attempt to increase the efficiency of screening by focusing on a small, high-risk segment of the general population (other than older women) is presently not feasible, since this would exclude the vast majority of women who develop breast cancer.

Nevertheless, certain risk factors have been identified that may provide insight into the genesis of breast cancer (Fig. 2.2). In general, they can be divided into factors that confer a highly, moderately, or slightly elevated risk in comparison with individuals who do not have the factor. For example, women born in North America or Europe are far more likely to develop breast cancer than are women born in Asia. A previous personal history of breast cancer or a familial history of breast cancer, especially in a first-degree relative (sister, mother), elevates the relative risk of developing

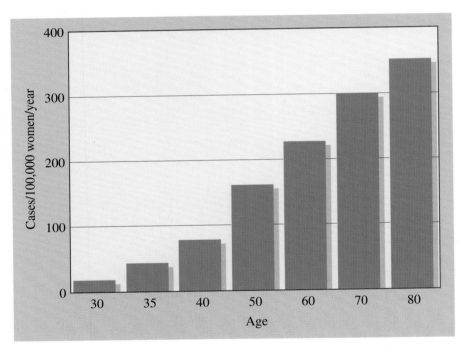

Figure 2.1 Age-specific incidence of breast cancer in the United States.

breast cancer over the individual's life by three- to fivefold. Some studies have suggested that this risk is higher in women whose sisters developed cancer under the age of 40, and the risk is further increased if their cancers were bilateral. In a few rare families, almost all women (and some men) develop breast cancer, often at an early age. Likewise, members of so-called familial cancer families, such as those with the Li–Fraumeni syndrome, have an extraordinarily high risk of developing breast cancer, as well as other epithelial and mesenchymal malignancies.

These apparently inherited patterns of disease have led to investigations of genetic alterations that may occur in patients who develop breast cancer. Two basic approaches to this goal have been used. In one, investigators try to associate (or link) the development of breast cancer in high-risk families with the expression of certain patterns of polymorphic genes at previously located chromosomal sites. These polymorphic sites may have no role in the development of the disease, but rather are geographically related (linked) to an unknown gene of interest. For example, if a certain genotype (such as a specific blood group antigen type) is consistently expressed by members of a family who have breast cancer but is randomly distributed among unaffected members, then the "breast cancer gene"

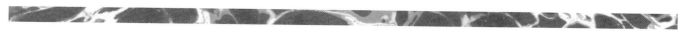

Figure 2.2 Breast Cancer Risk Factors

Highly Elevated Risk (relative risk at least 4 times that of population without factor)	Moderately Elevated Risk (Relative risk 2 to 4 times that of population without factor)	Slightly Elevated Risk (Relative risk 1 to 2 times that of population without factor)
Female	Any first degree relative with history of breast cancer	Moderate alcohol intake
Age > 50	Upper social/economic class	Menarche <12 years old
Country of birth in North America, Northern Europe	Prolonged uninterrupted menses (late first pregnancy, nulliparous)	? Hormonal replacement therapy
Personal history of prior breast cancer	Postmenopausal obesity	? Oral contraceptives
Family history bilateral, premenopausal, or familial cancer syndrome	Personal history of prior carcinoma of ovary or endometrium	? Diet
Atypical proliferative benign breast disease, especially with family history	Proliferative benign breast disease, if no atypia	

must be "linked" (located on the same chromosome) to the known gene (Fig. 2.3). If the genotype of the marker gene is randomly distributed among those individuals with or without breast cancer, then the genes are not linked. For example, recent data have implicated a gene present on chromosome 17. Once such a site

is identified, further studies are aimed at identifying the specific gene (and its product) involved in the development of the cancer.

A second approach has been to identify certain candidate genes that might be responsible for the development of cancers. These "oncogenes" can produce

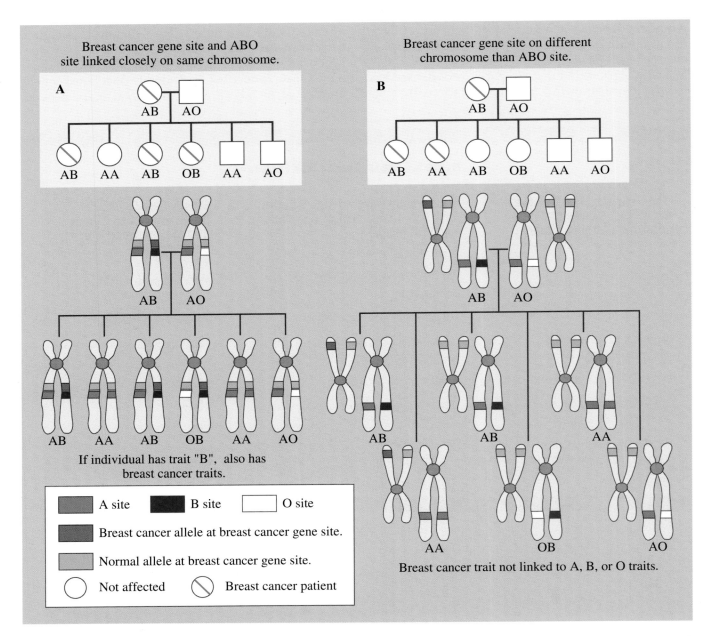

Figure 2.3 Example of linkage analysis. In family A, development of breast cancer is associated with expression of the "B" phenotype. This suggests that the gene responsible for breast cancer is geographically "linked" on the same chromosome as the polymorphic ABO gene, and therefore is not randomly segregated during meiosis. This linkage is schematically represented underneath the family pedigree. X = breast cancer allele at breast cancer gene

site; Y = normal allele at breast cancer gene site. In family B, development of breast cancer is not associated with expression of A, B, or O. This suggests that the breast cancer gene is located on a different chromosome from the ABO gene and segregates randomly during meiosis, as schematically illustrated underneath the family pedigree.

tumors in in vitro models and can be detected at a reasonably high frequency in primary cancer tissues. For the most part, oncogenes are actually derivatives of normal cellular genes, designated proto-oncogenes, which have been altered so that they function abnormally and cause malignant cell transformation. Oncogenes can be either dominant or recessive (Fig. 2.4). Dominant proto-oncogenes are normally involved in stimulating cell growth and/or inhibiting differentiation, and their function is regulated to ensure restricted growth in the appropriate setting (see Fig. 2.4A). The expression or function of these genes is altered, often by mutations at certain critical sites, so that they are no longer subject to normal control processes (see Fig. 2.4B). One dominant oncogene in breast cancer is the so-called HER-2/*neu* or c-*erbB2* gene. This proto-oncogene apparently encodes for a growth factor receptor, but amplification and/or over-

expression of the proto-oncogene by breast cancer cells appears to be associated with more aggressive behavior and poorer clinical outcome.

Recessive proto-oncogenes function normally as suppressors of growth or as stimulants of differentiation (Fig. 2.5). Deletions or "lethal" mutations at critical sites of these genes lead to constitutive activity of otherwise normal growth-promoting genes, resulting in unrestricted proliferation or lack of differentiation. It is important to note that both alleles of a recessive oncogene must be altered, in a so-called "two-hit" manner, to produce transformation (see Fig. 2.5C). Recent investigations have demonstrated that members of Li–Fraumeni families that develop breast cancer have inherited somatic mutations of one copy of the recessive oncogene designated p53, whereas both alleles of unaffected members are of the wild type. Therefore, a second mutation to the remaining copy presumably is

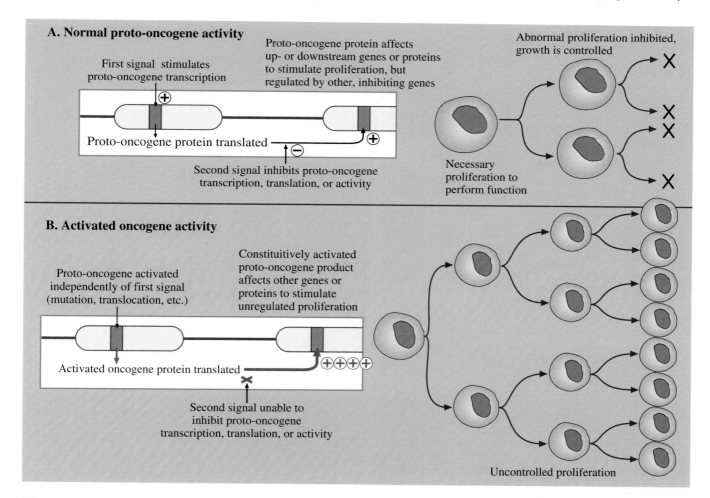

Figure 2.4 Dominant oncogenic changes. (A) A normal, proto-oncogene encodes for a protein that causes other genes or proteins to stimulate proliferation. However, expression of this gene or activity of its protein product is regulated by the activity of a sec-ond gene, resulting in controlled growth. In (B) the protooncogene has been activated, and expression of the gene or activity of its product is no longer subject to the inhibitory effects of the regulatory gene(s), leading to uncontrolled proliferation.

Risk Factors, Epidemiology, and Development of Breast Cancer

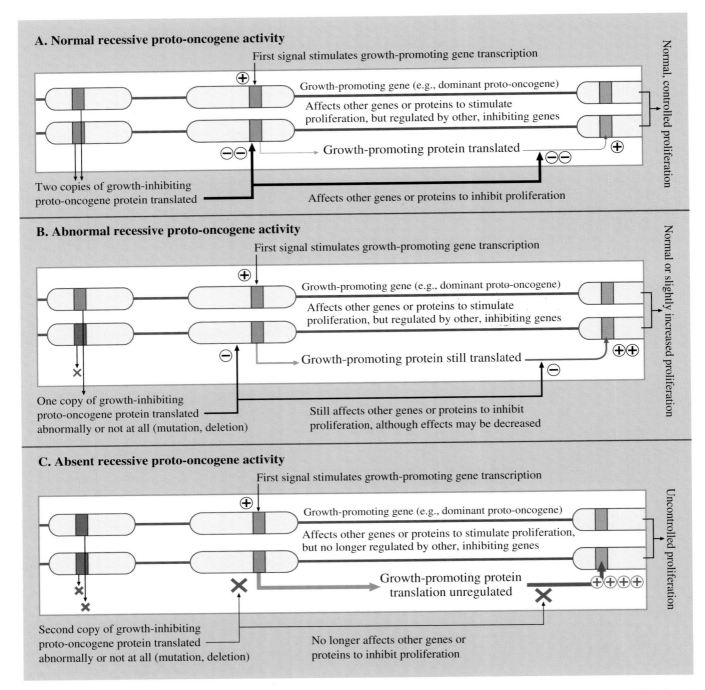

A. Normal recessive proto-oncogene activity

First signal stimulates growth-promoting gene transcription

Growth-promoting gene (e.g., dominant proto-oncogene)

Affects other genes or proteins to stimulate proliferation, but regulated by other, inhibiting genes

Growth-promoting protein translated

Two copies of growth-inhibiting proto-oncogene protein translated

Affects other genes or proteins to inhibit proliferation

Normal, controlled proliferation

B. Abnormal recessive proto-oncogene activity

First signal stimulates growth-promoting gene transcription

Growth-promoting gene (e.g., dominant proto-oncogene)

Affects other genes or proteins to stimulate proliferation, but regulated by other, inhibiting genes

Growth-promoting protein still translated

One copy of growth-inhibiting proto-oncogene protein translated abnormally or not at all (mutation, deletion)

Still affects other genes or proteins to inhibit proliferation, although effects may be decreased

Normal or slightly increased proliferation

C. Absent recessive proto-oncogene activity

First signal stimulates growth-promoting gene transcription

Growth-promoting gene (e.g., dominant proto-oncogene)

Affects other genes or proteins to stimulate proliferation, but no longer regulated by other, inhibiting genes

Growth-promoting protein translation unregulated

Second copy of growth-inhibiting proto-oncogene protein translated abnormally or not at all (mutation, deletion)

No longer affects other genes or proteins to inhibit proliferation

Uncontrolled proliferation

Figure 2.5 Recessive oncogenic changes. (A) The recessive proto-oncogene produces a protein product that serves to control other genes or proteins to control proliferation. (B) One copy of the recessive proto-oncogene has been altered (e.g., mutation, deletion, translocation), and now only one copy of the gene functions to control proliferation. (C) The remaining copy of the recessive proto-oncogene has been altered, resulting in elimination of its growth-inhibiting function and unregulated cell proliferation. The first alteration may be a somatic, inherited change, as occurs in certain familial cancers, or both alterations may occur at random after birth in the tissue from which the cancer originates.

sufficient to result in breast cancer. Studies are ongoing to determine if alterations in p53 or other recessive oncogenes are also involved in more common varieties of breast cancer.

These results do not imply that breast cancer is exclusively an inherited, genetic disease. In fact, considerable data exist indicating that exogenous factors may be as important as genetic causes. For example, "strong" risk factors include older age, prolonged, uninterrupted menses (late first pregnancy, nulliparity), country of origin (independent of ethnic background), and perhaps diet, alcohol intake, and use of estrogens (see Fig. 2.2). These observations suggest possible avenues of prevention, and investigative trials of lifestyle changes, diet modification, and/or chemoprevention with antiestrogen agents such as tamoxifen are under way.

Of interest is that most benign breast lesions are not associated with an increased risk of breast cancer. For example, fibroadenomas or cysts may mimic breast cancers clinically but are not "precursors" of malignancy. However, women with certain types of proliferative breast diseases have a three- to fivefold increased risk of developing breast cancer, which approaches tenfold if they have a strong family history (Fig. 2.6). Treatment recommendations are not necessarily more aggressive for these patients, but they should be followed closely. Laboratory and clinical studies of proliferative breast diseases may provide further insights into the step-by-step development of breast cancer.

It is probable that the genesis of breast cancer is multifactorial, with genetic, inherent metabolic, and environmental components. A reasonable model might include an inherited genetic susceptibility toward developing breast cancer (for example, inheritance of one or more abnormal recessive oncogenes) which, when coupled with exposure to a particular environmental factor (for example, something in the diet), leads to the development of a malignant clone of cells (Fig. 2.7). Subsequent uncontrolled growth, invasion, and metastases might then be the result of further exposure to factors that are not "oncogenic" per se but rather promote these behaviors in already transformed cells. These might include substances with growth-stimulating potential, such as estrogens. Other mutagenic factors might produce dominant but weak oncogenic changes that would be of no consequence in "normal" cells, but when coupled with prior recessive (or dominant) oncogenic mutations, as well as exposure to growth potentiators, might lead to the malignant phenotype. It has also been speculated that a variety of "anti-oncogenic" mechanisms have evolved to protect against the development of malignancy, such as programmed cell death in the event of an oncogenic mutation or immune surveillance with elimination of transformed cells. If these mechanisms do exist, the development of invasive, metastatic breast cancer must include oncogenic steps that evade such innate controls. The breast cancer model should also include satisfactory explanations for both the tissue specificity of

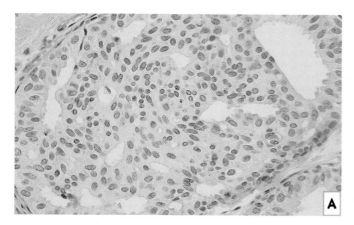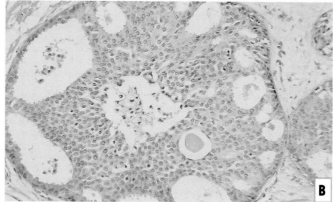

Figure 2.6 (A) Florid intraductal hyperplasia without atypia. This lesion is characterized by a proliferation of epithelial cells which fill and distend the involved duct. However, the cells vary in size, shape, and orientation. In addition, the secondary spaces produced by the cell proliferation tend to be elongated. Lesions such as this are associated with only a mildly elevated risk of breast cancer (i.e., 1.5–2-fold). (B) Atypical ductal hyperplasia. This proliferative lesion is considered "atypical" because it has some, but not all, of the features of ductal carcinoma in situ (DCIS). In contrast to florid hyperplasia without atypia, this lesion has a suspicious population of uniform cells with monotonous nuclei, raising the possibility of DCIS. However, there is also a population of polarized cells at the periphery of the duct, distinguishing this lesion from DCIS, which would lack this feature. Proliferative lesions such as this are associated with moderately elevated breast cancer risk (three- to fivefold).

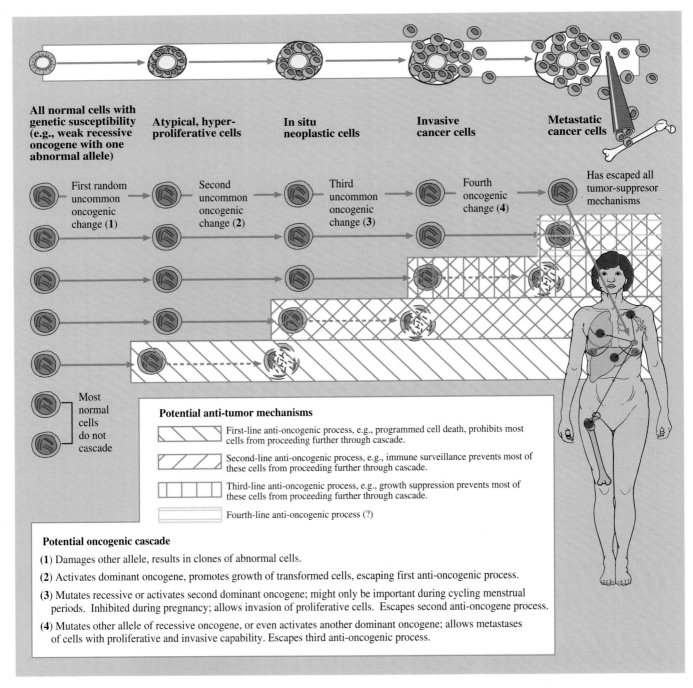

All normal cells with genetic susceptibility (e.g., weak recessive oncogene with one abnormal allele)

Atypical, hyper-proliferative cells

In situ neoplastic cells

Invasive cancer cells

Metastatic cancer cells

First random uncommon oncogenic change (1)

Second uncommon oncogenic change (2)

Third uncommon oncogenic change (3)

Fourth oncogenic change (4)

Has escaped all tumor-suppresor mechanisms

Most normal cells do not cascade

Potential anti-tumor mechanisms

First-line anti-oncogenic process, e.g., programmed cell death, prohibits most cells from proceeding further through cascade.

Second-line anti-oncogenic process, e.g., immune surveillance prevents most of these cells from proceeding further through cascade.

Third-line anti-oncogenic process, e.g., growth suppression prevents most of these cells from proceeding further through cascade.

Fourth-line anti-oncogenic process (?)

Potential oncogenic cascade

(1) Damages other allele, results in clones of abnormal cells.

(2) Activates dominant oncogene, promotes growth of transformed cells, escaping first anti-oncogenic process.

(3) Mutates recessive or activates second dominant oncogene; might only be important during cycling menstrual periods. Inhibited during pregnancy; allows invasion of proliferative cells. Escapes second anti-oncogene process.

(4) Mutates other allele of recessive oncogene, or even activates another dominant oncogene; allows metastases of cells with proliferative and invasive capability. Escapes third anti-oncogenic process.

Figure 2.7 Hypothetical model of breast cancer development and progression. A subject with a genetic susceptibility to breast cancer (for example, mutation of one copy of a weak recessive oncogene) is exposed to a random, uncommon factor that damages the other allele. This change might be insufficient to produce a malignant cell but results in a clone of abnormal cells (for example, atypical proliferative cells). Exposure of these cells to a second uncommon factor (for example, a dietary factor) results in a dominant but weak oncogenic change. This factor might not produce any change in cells that that do not contain prior recessive oncogenic changes. Exposure to a third factor (dominant or reces-sive), which by itself may be only weakly oncogenic, results in a combination of changes that produce a malignant cell. This factor might be oncogenic only during certain periods of life in which other promoting factors are present or tumor-inhibiting factors are decreased (for example, in women with continued, uninterrupted menstrual cycles). A variety of mechanisms may exist to prevent progression of oncogenesis, including immune surveillance, pro-grammed cell death, as well as genetic growth control ("recessive oncogene"). The effects of each mechanism may be more or less important during different stages of oncogenesis.

oncogenic factors and the critical effect of timing of the exposures (for example, an early full-term pregnancy appears to be protective, whereas a late one is not).

In summary, present knowledge does not reliably identify a high-risk subgroup (other than older women) in whom screening should be focused. Nor do we have sufficient insight into environmental causes of breast cancer to suggest lifestyle changes that might lead to prevention of breast cancer. Nevertheless, research in the areas of both inherited and environmental oncogenesis is proceeding rapidly and may provide effective approaches to these problems in the near future.

SUGGESTED READING

Ames B. (1983) Dietary carcinogens and anticarcinogens: oxygen radicals and degenerative diseases. *Science* 221:1256–1263.

Dupont W, Page D. (1985) Risk factors for breast cancer in women with proliferative breast disease. *N Engl J Med* 312:146–151.

Hall J, Lee M, Newman B, et al. (1990) Linkage of early-onset familial breast cancer to chromosome 17q21. *Science* 250:1684–1689.

Henderson B, Ross R, Bernstein L. (1988) Estrogens as a cause of human cancer: the Richard and Hinda Rosenthal Foundation Award Lecture. *Cancer Res* 48:246–253.

Henderson IC. (1990) What can a woman do about her risk of dying of breast cancer? *Curr Probl Cancer* 4.

Hulka B. (1990) Hormone-replacement therapy and the risk of breast cancer. *CA* 40:289–296.

Kelsey J, Berkowitz G. (1988) Breast cancer epidemiology. *Cancer Res* 48:5615–5623.

Li F, Fraumeni J. (1982) Prospective study of a family cancer syndrome. *JAMA* 247:2692–2694.

Lynch H, Watson P, Conway T, Lynch J. (1990) Clinical/genetic features in hereditary breast cancer. *Breast Cancer Res Treat* 15:63–71.

Malkin D, Li F, Strong L, et al. (1990) Germ line p53 mutations in a familial syndrome of breast cancer. *Science* 255:1233–1238.

Ottman R, King M-K, Pike M, Henderson B. (1983) Practical guide for estimating risk for familial breast cancer. *Lancet* 2:556–558.

Slamon D, Clark G, Wong S, Levin W, Ullrich A, McGuire W. (1987) Human breast cancer: Correlation of relapse and survival with amplification of the HER-2/*neu* oncogene. *Science* 235:177–182.

Willett W. (1989) The search for the causes of breast and colon cancer. *Nature* 338:389–394.

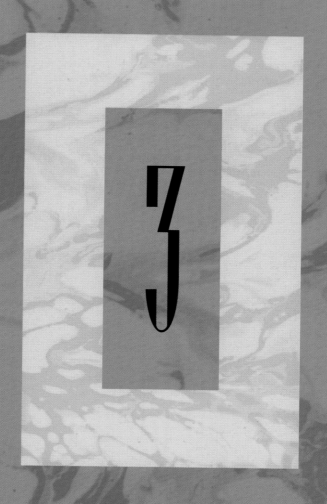

Normal Anatomy
and Development

Stuart J. Schnitt

The normal adult female breast is composed of an admixture of epithelial and stromal elements. The epithelial elements consist of a series of branching ducts which connect the structural and functional units of the breast, the lobules, to the nipple (Fig. 3.1). The stroma is composed of variable amounts of adipose tissue and fibrous connective tissue, and comprises the majority of the breast volume in the nonlactational state.

At birth, the epithelial component of the breast consists of a small number of rudimentary branching ducts beneath the nipple–areola complex. During the prepubertal years these ducts exhibit relatively slow but progressive growth and branching. In males, breast development ceases at this stage. At the time of puberty in the female there is increased growth and branching of the ducts, accompanied by an increase in the stromal component. In the postpubertal years, the ter-

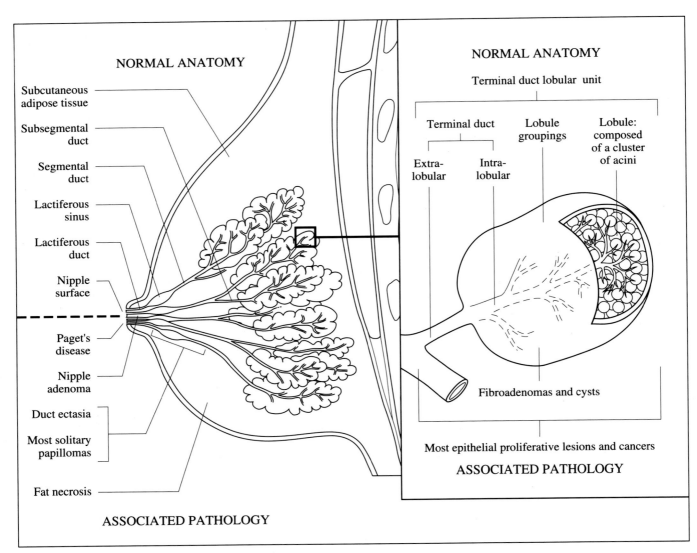

Figure 3.1 Diagram of breast anatomy. The epithelial component of the breast is organized into lobules, which are composed of clusters of acini. These feed into the terminal ducts, which in turn coalesce to form larger ducts. There are about 15–20 large ducts which terminate at the nipple. The epithelial elements are supported by a stroma consisting of fat and fibrous tissue. The presumed sites of origin of several pathologic conditions that affect the breast are also illustrated in the figure. (Adapted from Hayes, 1991).

minal ducts give rise to sacular buds, but continued stromal growth accounts for most of the increase in breast volume during this time. During pregnancy many secretory glands develop from each bud. By the end of pregnancy the glandular component has increased to the point where the breast is composed primarily of epithelial elements, with relatively little stroma. These changes persist during lactation. In the postlactational state there is glandular atrophy and decreased breast size. The stroma once again becomes the predominant component of the breast. However, the epithelial components do not regress completely, and the glandular elements remain more prominent than in the virginal breast. After menopause there is atrophy of the glandular elements, with a marked diminution in the number of lobules. In some areas of the breast lobules disappear completely, and only ducts remain. The fibrous connective tissue component of the stroma also diminishes, whereas stromal adipose tissue accumulation increases.

The histologic features of the normal breast are illustrated in Figure 3.2 through 3.6

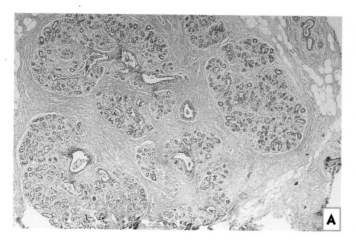

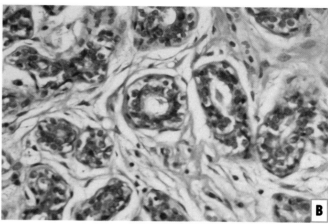

Figure 3.2 (A) Low-power photomicrograph of normal adult female breast tissue, demonstrating several lobules and a few extralobular ducts. Each lobule consists of a cluster of small glands, the acini, which feed into a terminal duct. Together, these structures define the terminal duct lobular unit. Note that the lobules are invested with loose, fibrous connective tissue stroma, demarcating them from the surrounding extralobular stroma which is composed of more dense connective tissue. (B) High-power view of several acini of a lobule. The acini have a single layer of cuboidal epithelial cells (closer to the lumen). Beneath this epithelium is a layer of myoepithelial cells which often have clear cytoplasm. The lobules show subtle histologic variations during the different phases of the menstrual cycle.

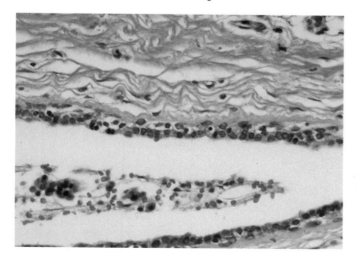

Figure 3.3 This extralobular duct, like the acini, exhibits an inner (luminal) layer of cuboidal epithelial cells and outer layer of myoepithelial cells. In this section the myoepithelial layer appears discontinuous.

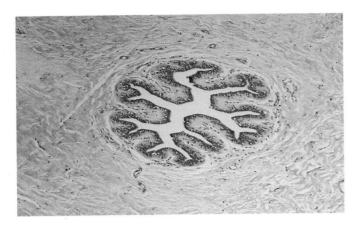

Figure 3.4 The irregular, pleated contour of this duct is typical of ducts present beneath the nipple.

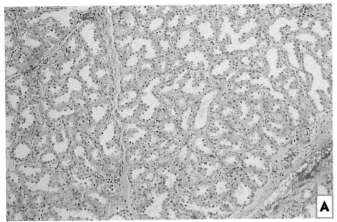

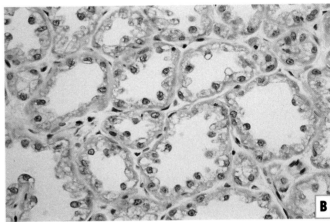

Figure 3.5 Lactational change. (A) Low-power of breast showing lactational change. Many secretory glands comprise the bulk of the breast tissue; intervening connective tissue is minimal. (B) Higher-power photomicrograph showing several secretory glands. The cytoplasm of the epithelial cells is vacuolated. Some of the nuclei bulge into the gland lumens, imparting a "hobnail" appearance to the cells.

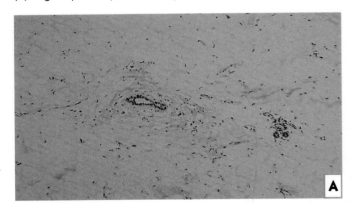

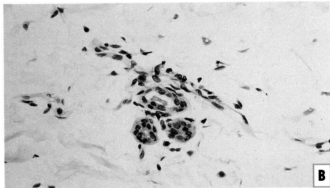

Figure 3.6 Atrophy. This is a section of breast tissue from a postmenopausal woman. The stroma is composed primarily of adipose tissue. (A) At low power a single duct and an atrophic lobule are evident. (B) Higher-power view of atrophic lobule.

REFERENCES

Azzopardi JG. (1979) *Problems in Breast Pathology.* Philadelphia: WB Saunders, 8–22

Haagensen CD. (1986) *Disease of the Breast*, 3rd ed. Philadelphia: WB Saunders, 1–55.

Hayes DF. (1991) Breast cancer. In Skarin AT, ed. *Atlas of Diagnostic Oncology.* New York: Gower Medical Publishing, 6.1–6.31.

Page DL, Anderson TJ. (1987) *Diagnostic Histopathology of the Breast.* Edinburgh: Churchill Livingstone, 4–29.

Vogel PM, Georgiade NG, Fetter BF, Vogel FS, McCarty KS. (1981) The correlation of histologic changes in the human breast with the menstrual cycle. *Am J Pathol* 104:23–34.

4

Mammography

Paul C. Stomper

MORTALITY REDUCTION IN BREAST CANCER ACHIEVED BY SCREENING MAMMOGRAPHY: THE SCREENING TRIALS

Several large prospective trials have been performed in which tens of thousands of women were randomized to either (1) intensive breast screening programs, including routine mammography and physical exam or routine mammography alone, or (2) routine follow-up according to their physician's discretion. Overall, the results of these studies suggested that mammography screening is associated with an approximately 20 to 30 percent reduction in breast cancer mortality in women age 50 and older. Case-controlled studies in which populations of women who had 100 percent compliance for screening mammography were compared with a population of women who had not undergone mammography show a reduction in mortality of 50 percent or more.

Earlier, several uncontrolled trials demonstrated that screening mammography leads to detection of breast cancer at an earlier stage than physical exam, but these studies did not prove that such earlier detection was linked to a prolonged survival time. Early detection of the disease means, by definition, that patients will live longer from their time of diagnosis (lead-time bias). They may not, however, live longer than they would have otherwise, unless therapy initiated at the time of early detection is more effective than therapy given at a later time. The randomized, controlled screening trials demonstrate that the apparent benefits of screening mammography, as suggested by the noncontrolled trials, are not due merely to lead-time bias but to a true reduction in mortality by early treatment (Fig. 4.1).

SCREENING RECOMMENDATIONS

The American Cancer Society recommendation includes annual physical examination beginning at age 40 and screening mammography at one- to two-year intervals between the ages of 40 and 50 and every year at age 50 and older. Consideration should be given to earlier mammographic screening for women considered at high risk, that is, those with a family history of breast cancer, previous breast biopsy demonstrating atypical ductal hyperplasia, or prior breast cancer.

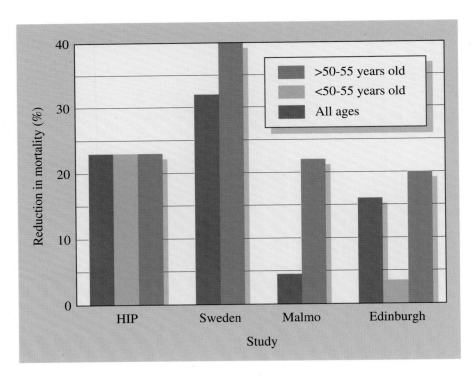

Figure 4.1 Relative reduction in mortality in woman screened for early breast cancer in randomized trials. [Sources: HIP, Health Plan of New York., from Chu, Smart, and Tarone (1988); Sweden, from Tabar, Gad, Holmberg, et al. (1985): Malmö, Sweden, from Andersson, Aspegren, Janzon, et al. (1988); Edinburgh, Scotland, from Roberts, Alexander, Anderson, et al. (1990).]

COMPLEMENTARY ROLES OF MAMMOGRAPHY AND PHYSICAL EXAMINATION

More than 90 percent of all breast cancers that are detected by annual screening with mammography and physical examination are identified by mammography. In the BCDDP (Breast Cancer Detection Demonstration Project), 42 percent of cancers were detected by mammography alone (Fig. 4.2). Approximately 85 percent of BCDDP cancers in women of ages 40 to 49 were seen on mammography as compared with 93 percent in women of age 50 and older. This is most likely related to the obscuration of noncalcified soft tissue malignancies by increased parenchymal density in younger breasts. Even in uniformly dense breasts, present in 41 percent of women age 49 and younger and in 18 percent of women age 50 and older in several series, most early breast cancers are still detectable on mammography as microcalcifications or areas of architectural distortion of dense tissue.

Physical examination is complementary to mammography. Clinically palpable cancers can be detected in patients with normal mammograms, usually those with dense breast tissue. With only a few exceptions, neither a normal mammogram nor a normal physical exam should diminish the level of suspicion raised by an abnormality of the other.

TECHNIQUE

High-quality mammography requires dedicated mammographic equipment and radiologic technologists with special training in mammography. At present, film-screen mammography is the predominant technique used in both the United States and Europe. High-resolution equipment with small focal spot sizes, short exposure time, and long source-to-image distances are needed to resolve structures of 150 μm and even smaller (e.g., microcalcifications) for the detection of early breast cancers. In addition, magnification x-ray technique, which can resolve microcalcifications as small as 40 μm, is helpful as an aid in the characterization and assessment of extent of microcalcification clusters.

Film-screen mammography uses x-ray exposure of a high-resolution film adjacent to a fluorescent screen to create the breast image. Magnification technique uses a small focal spot and an increased object-to-film distance for improved resolution. Film-screen mammography requires compression of the breast between the

Figure 4.2 Mode of Detection of Breast Cancer During Screening in BCDDP Study*

	40-49	50-59
Mammography only	36%	42%
Mammography and physical examination	50%	50%
Physical examination only	13%	7%

*From Baker (1982), with permission.

parallel plastic compression plate and the underlying film-screen cassette holder during the x-ray exposure. Compression enhances resolution by improving clarity and improving image contrast by diminishing scatter radiation and permitting uniform exposure (Fig. 4.3). By spreading the glandular tissue apart and holding the breast away from the chest wall, it markedly increases diagnostic information on the image. A multicenter survey of more than 1,800 women demonstrated that 88 percent of women experience only mild discomfort or none during the mammogram and that severe discomfort or pain was an uncommon occurrence. Physical discomfort did not cause any woman to reconsider having another mammogram.

The radiation dose from film-screen mammography ranges from approximately 100 to 400 millirads (0.1 to 0.4 rads) midglandular absorbed dose for two-view examination of the breast. Recent review and extrapolation from high-dose data suggest that the radiation risk is age-related and appears negligible, if present at all, in women of ages 35 and older.

MAMMOGRAPHIC FEATURES OF BREAST CANCER

Breast cancer exhibits a range of mammographic appearances. However, significant overlap in the mammographic appearance between cancers and many benign entities exists because they are frequently similar in gross morphology. Nonetheless, there are two general categories for mammographic indications of malignancy: (1) soft tissue masses, or (2) clustered microcalcifications—calcium particles of various size and shape measuring 100 microns to 1 mm in diameter and numbering greater than 4–5 per cubic cm.

A spiculated soft-tissue mass is the most specific mammographic feature of malignancy, with an almost 99 percent chance of representing cancer (Figs. 4.4 and 4.5). Approximately one-third of noncalcified cancers appear as spiculated masses. About 25 percent appear as irregularly outlined masses, 25 percent as less specific round, oval, or lobulated masses with indistinct borders, and less than 10 percent present as well-defined round, oval, or lobulated masses. Well-defined solid masses are associated with a 0 to 7 percent pre-

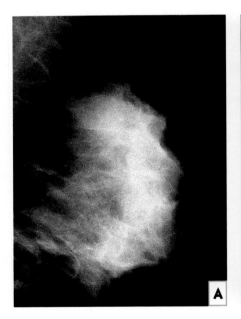
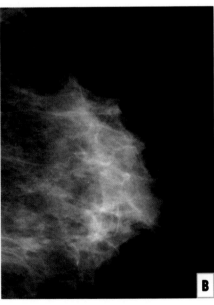

Figure 4.3 Film-screen mammogram technique. (A) Oblique projection obtained with poor breast compression creates an overall increase in density and potential for obscuration of lesions. (B) A mammogram obtained immediately after A with proper compression technique exhibits greater detail and potential for detection of small lesions. Compression until the breast skin becomes taut is an important component of film-screen technique but need not be painful for most women.

dictive value for malignancy in several series. Short interval (six-month, then annually) mammographic follow-up of small, well-defined nodules is considered appropriate management. Of note is that a variety of benign nodules may be observed with mammography. Examples of such a finding which do not require short-interval follow-up include intramammary or even low axillary lymph nodes. Approximately 5 percent of non-calcified cancers present as areas of architectural distortion of dense tissue.

Microcalcifications are seen in approximately 60 percent of cancers detected by mammography (Figs. 4.6 and 4.7). Histologically, these represent intraductal calcifications in areas of necrotic tumor, usually comedocarcinoma, or calcifications of mucin-secreting tumors such as the cribriform or micropapillary subtype of intraductal cancer. Linear, branching microcalcifications usually associated with comedocarcinoma have a higher predictive value for malignancy than granular microcalcifications, that is, nonlinear, irregular calcifi-

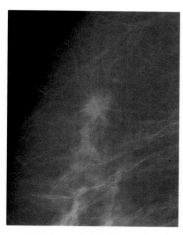

Figure 4.4 Stage I (T_1N_0) breast cancer. Magnified view of a mammogram from a 50-year-old woman with a history of "lumpy" breasts shows a 1-cm spiculated mass in the superior portion of the breast. The lesion was excised and was found to be an invasive ductal carcinoma.

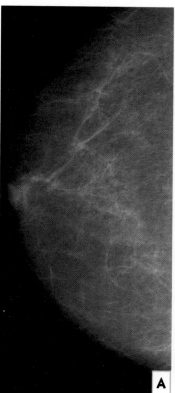
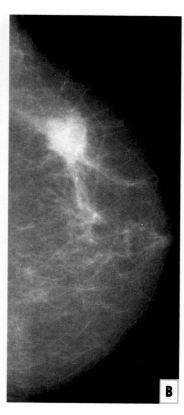

Figure 4.5 Stage IIA (T_2N_0) breast cancer. (A,B) Mammogram from a 65-year-old woman shows a 2.5-cm stellate mass in the upper outer quadrant of the right breast which was easily palpated. Histologic examination after resection identified this as an invasive ductal carcinoma.

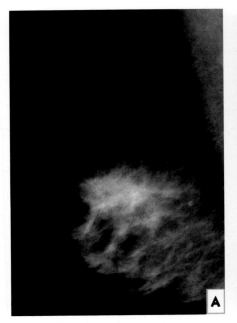

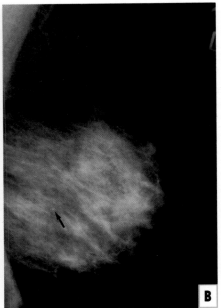

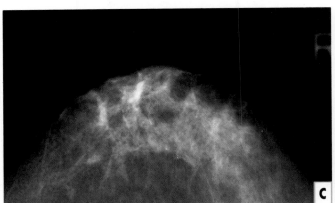

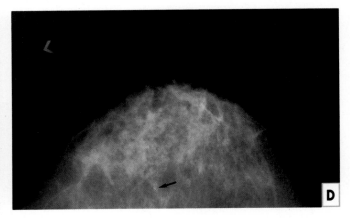

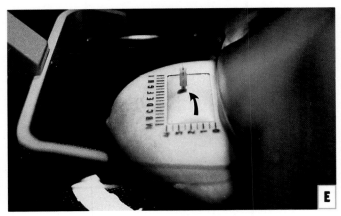

Figure 4.6 Detection of suspicious microcalcifications by screening mammography and localization for biopsy. This screening mammogram in an asymptomatic 55-year-old woman detected a 3-mm microcalcification cluster *(arrow)* in the left breast which raised suspicion for malignancy. (A) Right medial-lateral oblique projection. (B) Left medial-lateral oblique projection. (C) Right craniocaudad projection. (D) Left craniocaudad projection. (E) Another patient undergoing film-screen mammogram during needle localization procedure in which hookwire needle *(arrow)* is placed within the grid-coordinate aperture in the plastic compression device.

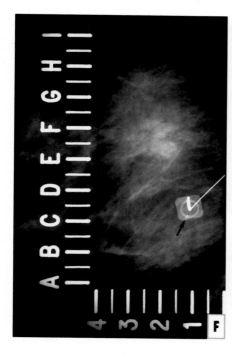

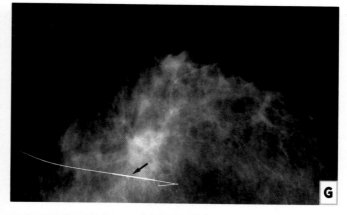

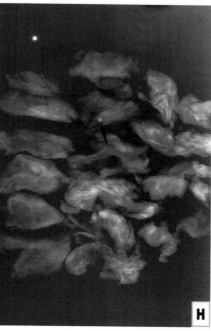

Figure 4.6, continued (F) Needle localization procedure. Lateral view of patient in (B) shows the needle placement through the opening in the grid coordinate compression plate so that the needle was adjacent to microcalcifications (*arrow*). (G) The craniocaudad view obtained at the end of the needle localization procedure shows the final position of the hookwire needle. The 3-mm microcalcification cluster was just posterior to the thick segment of the hookwire (*arrow*). (H) Specimen radiography after sectioning. After specimen radiography of the entire specimen, the specimen was sectioned by the pathologist and re-radiographed to further direct the pathologist to the small area of calcifications (*arrow*), which was shown to represent ductal carcinoma in situ.

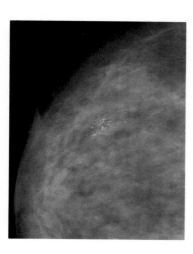

Figure 4.7 Stage I (T_1N_2) breast cancer. Magnification projection of a 52-year-old asymptomatic woman demonstrates the classic indeterminate clustered microcalcifications of several shapes and sizes, highly suggestive of carcinoma. Some exhibit linear branching, which is even more suggestive of a ductal lesion. Biopsy confirmed an early invasive ductal carcinoma.

cations of varying size and shape. However, a slight majority of mammographically detected cancers associated with microcalcifications exhibit the granular type. Benign calcifications that are not suspicious for malignancy include vascular calcifications, skin calcifications, rim-like calcifications, large coarse calcifications, and smooth round or oval calcifications (Figs. 4.8, 4.9, 4.10, and 4.11).

Ductal carcinoma in situ (DCIS) comprises 25 to 56 percent of clinically occult cancers detected by mammography in several published series. Since there is no mammographic feature of ductule basement membrane invasion, it is not possible to distinguish the pure intraductal from the infiltrating ductal type of carcinoma on the basis of the mammographic appearance. Approximately 70 percent of occult breast cancers presenting as microcalcifications only and 15 percent of breast cancers presenting as noncalcified soft-tissue abnormalities only are intraductal cancers.

PREDICTIVE VALUE OF MAMMOGRAPHY

Large series of needle localization procedures for clinically occult lesions reported from American referral hospitals show a positive predictive value of mammography of 20 to 30 percent (predictive value is defined as the number of cancers detected divided by the total number of biopsies performed for clinically occult lesions deemed suspicious by the mammographer). This percentage will increase as more American women undergo follow-up or incident screening, providing the mammographer with "baseline" mammograms for com-

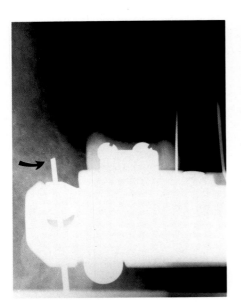

Figure 4.8 Stereotactic fine-needle aspiration of suspicious microcalcifications (*arrow*). Cytologic diagnosis of clinically occult breast malignancy, especially with microcalcifications, is associated with a false-negative rate of approximately 5 percent. Excisional biopsy is usually recommended for diagnosis of any suspicious mammographic finding.

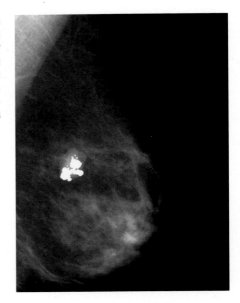

Figure 4.9 Evaluation of calcifications. Oblique mammogram demonstrates a classic benign, partially calcified fibroadenoma with typical coarse, popcorn-like calcifications. These findings are not suspicious and do not require biopsy.

parison, as is the case for most women in the Swedish screening trials in which predictive values of up to 70 percent have been suggested. Threshold for biopsy is also affected by the health care environment and the expectations of women being screened. Several series or biopsies for clinically palpable abnormalities also show a positive predictive value of 20 to 30 percent.

The most commonly used method in the United States for accurate guidance for the biopsy of nonpal- pable abnormalities is the mammographically guided hookwire needle localization technique (see Figs. 4.6 and 4.8). Specimen radiography of the excised tissue is then mandatory to confirm the accurate removal of the mammographic abnormality and to guide the pathologist to the area of the lesion for histologic sampling. Specimen radiography is accurate for the identification of both noncalcified and calcified lesions (see Fig. 4.6).

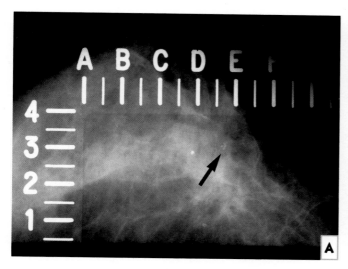

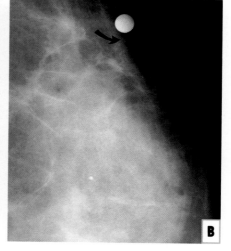

Figure 4.10 (A) Evaluation of skin calcifications. Craniocaudad mammogram with the grid coordinate localization compression plate in a 54-year-old woman demonstrated a 5-mm area of calcifications (arrow) which were deemed suspicious by a screening mammographer and were sent to a multidisciplinary breast center for needle localization and biopsy. (B) A tangential view with a B-B marker placed on the skin demonstrated that these calcifications represented benign dermal calcifications (arrow). Dermal calcifications are benign and characteristically have smooth, round, or oval margins and central lucency. Any calcifications with this suggestive appearance near the periphery of the breast should be differentiated from skin calcifications with appropriate skin marker localization techniques before a potentially disfiguring and unrewarding excisional biopsy of parenchymal tissue is attempted.

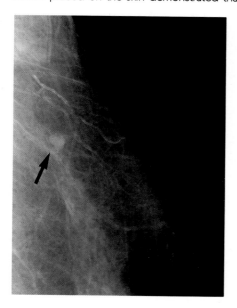

Figure 4.11 Benign intramammary lymph node. A well-circumscribed benign 6-mm nodule most likely represents a benign intramammary lymph node. These are characterized by their location in the upper outer aspect of the breast and the suggestion of a hilar notch. Routine mammographic follow-up is recommended. For other small, well-circumscribed, benign-appearing nodules, a six-month follow-up mammogram is considered appropriate management because of the widespread prevalence of such nodules and the very low (less than 1 to 2 percent) incidence of malignancy. Suggestion of growth on any follow-up mammogram warrants biopsy.

Fine-needle aspiration and core biopsy of clinically occult mammographic abnormalities are presently under investigation. Ultrasound-guided aspiration of indeterminate fluid-filled lesions and well-circumscribed masses of low predictive value can reduce the number of benign biopsies (Fig. 4.12). Stereotactic, mammographically guided fine-needle aspiration is associated with a false-negative rate of approximately 5 percent (see Fig. 4.8). Consequently, most suspicious mammographic lesions must be excised for histologic examination.

OTHER BREAST IMAGING MODALITIES

Ultrasound is a complementary tool to mammography and physical examination to differentiate cysts from solid masses (Figs. 4.12 and 4.13). Simple cysts by strict ultrasound criteria need no further intervention (Fig. 4.14). Indeterminate cysts may be aspirated under ultrasound guidance. Ultrasound may also be the initial diagnostic exam in a young patient with a well-circumscribed solid mass, which is most likely a benign fibroadenoma (see Fig. 4.13). Transillumination or

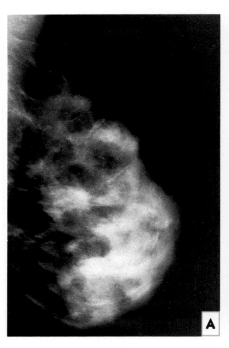
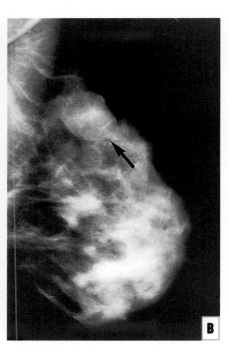
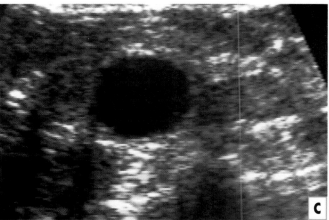

Figure 4.12 Complementary role of ultrasound in the evaluation of rounded masses. (A) Moderately dense breast tissue without evidence of malignancy on a screening mammogram performed on a 44-year-old woman. (B) Mammogram one year later demonstrated development of a partially obscured, rounded mass (arrow) in the upper aspect of the breast. (C) 7.5 mHz ultrasound examination performed with a hand-held transducer demonstrated the classic findings of a benign simple cyst, that is, smooth walls, lack of dependent echoes (distinguishing reverberation artifact near the skin surface), strong back-wall echo, and enhanced through-transmission. Ultrasound-guided fine-needle aspiration can be performed for indeterminate cysts (i.e., masses that have some but not all criteria for a simple cyst).

diaphanography (light scanning) is ineffective for the detection of clinically occult breast cancer. Magnetic resonance imaging and digital mammography remain investigational. CT is helpful for visualization and localization of deep lesions near the chest wall.

MAMMOGRAPHIC STAGING AND FOLLOW-UP OF THE PATIENT UNDERGOING BREAST-CONSERVING THERAPY

Mammography should be performed before any form of breast surgery and as part of the staging of any patient with the diagnosis of in situ or invasive breast cancer who is being considered for breast-conserving therapy. Magnification imaging of the region of the primary excision site in the post-biopsy breast is important to identify and assess the extent of residual tumor, especially microcalcifications (Fig. 4.15). However, lack of mammographic evidence of residual tumor does not exclude the presence of histologic tumor.

Proper mammographic follow-up of the irradiated breast is important to detect early, curable local recurrences and to avoid unnecessary biopsies and creation of anxiety in the patient being followed (Fig. 4.16). In one series of patients undergoing follow-up with both physi-

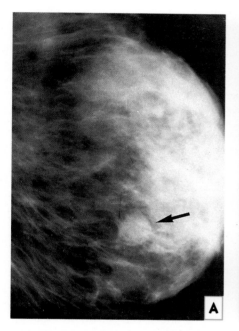

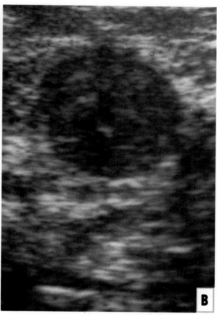

Figure 4.13 Evaluation of masses in young women. (A) Oblique mammogram demonstrates a predominantly well-circumscribed 2-cm mass in a 32-year-old woman. (B) 7.5 mHz ultrasound examination demonstrates a solid mass characterized by diffuse internal echoes and lack of strong back-wall echo or enhanced through-transmission. Although this appearance most commonly represents a benign fibroadenoma in a patient of this age, the possibility of malignancy cannot be excluded by the ultrasound appearance. Excisional biopsy was recommended and demonstrated a malignant lesion.

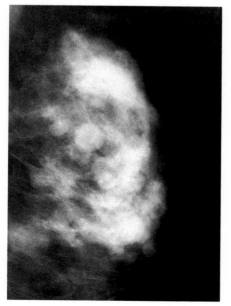

Figure 4.14 Evaluation of masses in young women. Multiple partially obscured, benign-appearing masses amid heterogeneous tissue in a 43-year-old woman. This appearance on a screening exam is most consistent with multiple benign cysts. Careful clinical and mammographic follow-up is performed. Ultrasound and/or cyst aspiration can be performed if there is suspicious change in one of the masses.

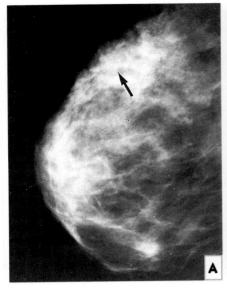
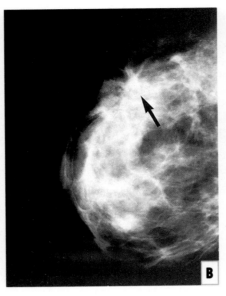
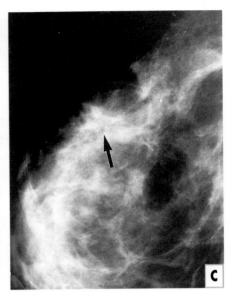

Figure 4.15 Evaluation and re-excision biopsy in a woman desiring breast-conserving therapy. (A) Mammogram shows a 15-mm cluster of microcalcifications which raised suspicion for malignancy (arrow). Needle localization and excisional biopsy were performed. Histologic evaluation demonstrated ductal carcinoma in situ. The patient preferred breast-conserving therapy if possible. (B) The postbiopsy mammogram revealed architectural distortion at the excision site and suggested several residual calcifications. (C) A postbiopsy magnification view of the excision site better demonstrated a 5-mm area of residual microcalcifications which would require excision before any form of breast-conserving therapy. Re-excision was performed and revealed residual in situ carcinoma with clean margins.

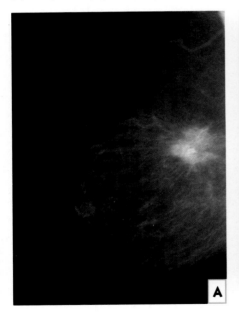
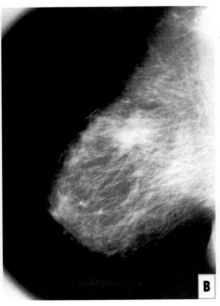
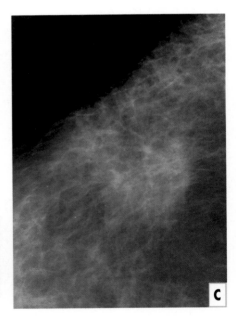

Figure 4.16 Serial mammography after breast-conserving primary therapy. This 53-year-old woman presented with a 2-cm infiltrating ductal carcinoma manifested as microcalcifications on a screening mammogram. This was excised with negative histologic margins and she received radiation therapy to the breast postoperatively. (A) Postbiopsy mammogram performed after complete excision of microcalcifications associated with invasive ductal carcinoma. Marked architectural distortion is seen at the excision site, a finding that should not raise concern on the postoperative baseline study. (B) Six-month postradiation treatment mammogram demonstrated benign radiation changes of skin thickening, increased parenchymal density, and overall breast retraction. This mammogram will serve as the patient's "new" baseline, against which future mammograms will be compared. (C) Routine magnification view of the primary excision site is obtained to increase sensitivity for detection of local recurrences in patients treated with breast-conserving therapy. A majority of local recurrences occur at or near the primary excision site.

cal exam and mammography, 35 percent of recurrent cancers in the irradiated breast were detected by mammography only (Figs. 4.17 and 4.18). The recurrences detected by mammography were more likely to be purely noninvasive than those detected by physical examination. Benign mammographic changes consisting of breast retraction, increased parenchymal density, skin thickening, development of coarse dystrophic calcifications or suture calcifications, and the presence of a mass or architectural distortion at the biopsy or hematoma site must be differentiated from recurrent cancer.

For patients who have undergone breast-conserving therapy, we perform routine mammographic follow-up at six months, 12 months, and every year subsequently (see Fig. 4.16).

SPECIAL CONSIDERATIONS

Silicone implants have been used for breast augmentation in several million women in the United States. The risks of these implants are controversial. Although few data are available, some reports have suggested an increase in cancers and in autoimmune phenomena in women who have undergone silicone implant augmentation. These controversies notwithstanding, silicone implants do complicate routine screening for early malignancy, since they are radiopaque and therefore obscure breast tissue during mammography. However, with specialized techniques, high-quality mammograms can be obtained in such women (Fig. 4.19).

Nipple discharge is a relatively common occurrence and is usually due to a benign process, such as ectasia,

Figure 4.17 Mode of Detection of Recurrent Cancer in Irradiated Breasts*

Mammogram only	35%
Physical examination only	39%
Both	26%

*From Stomper, Recht, Berenberg, et al. (1987), with permission.

Figure 4.18 Mammographic Appearances of Recurrent Cancer in Irradiated Breasts*

Calcifications	43%
Calcifications with a mass	29%
Mass or architectural distortion	21%
Inflammatory changes	7%

*From Stomper, Recht, Berenberg, et al. (1987), with permission.

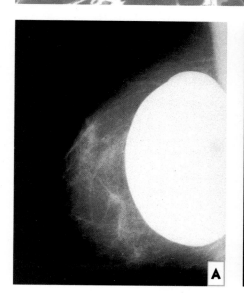
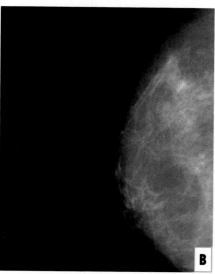

Figure 4.19 Evaluation of breasts after silicone implant augmentation. (A) Standard oblique projection of a breast containing a silicone implant inserted for breast augmentation. Although some parenchyma was visible, most of the breast was obscured by the implant. (B) An accessory projection of the same breast was obtained to better image the breast tissue around the implant by pulling the breast tissue away from the implant and including only that tissue within the compression plate and film-screen cassette. The presence of a breast implant, however, is still associated with some decrease in sensitivity of breast cancer detection by mammography.

papilloma, or fibrocystic changes. Further evaluation to distinguish these from malignancy should be initiated if the discharge is unilateral, occurs spontaneously (independent of nipple stimulation), is intermittent, and/or contains blood (although it should be noted that most bloody discharges are not malignant). Evaluation should include a careful history and physical exam searching for underlying breast masses, a mammogram, and in certain selected cases a ductogram (Fig. 4.20). If malignancy is suspected, workup and treatment should be performed in the appropriate manner. However, even benign nipple discharge may require surgical therapy, which involves terminal duct excision.

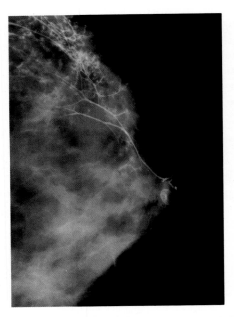

Figure 4.20 Ductogram or galactogram demonstrates opacification of a major areolar duct, distal terminal duct, and lobular network. Ductograms are performed by cannulation of a dilated major areolar duct and injection of a very small amount of iodinated contrast. Ductograms may be performed for some patients with bloody nipple discharge. Filling defects or blockages are nonspecific and may represent inspissation of secretions, benign papillomas, or malignancy. Some surgeons have used the ductogram to guide circumareolar excision of the dilated duct associated with nipple discharge for diagnosis. However, at present most surgeons locate, dissect, and excise a dilated central duct without ductogram guidance.

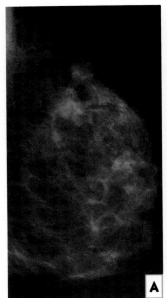
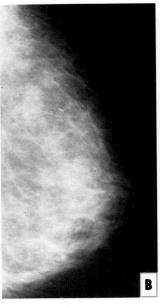
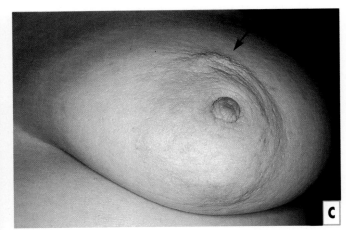

Figure 4.21 Stage IIIB (T4) breast cancer. A 35-year-old woman had a normal baseline mammogram (A). Seven months later she developed skin thickening and erythema of the breast (B,C). At that time her mammogram demonstrated a diffuse increase in density and skin thickening—characteristic findings in inflammatory breast cancer. Biopsy confirmed the diagnosis of inflammatory breast cancer. Arrow shows erythermatous blush, indicating inflammation. (From Hayes, 1991.)

MAMMOGRAPHIC STAGING AND FOLLOW-UP OF PATIENTS WITH LOCALLY ADVANCED PRIMARY BREAST CANCER

As noted, screening mammography is used to detect small, clinically inapparent lesions. In addition, mammography can also be very helpful in evaluating patients with palpable stage III breast cancer. For patients who present with locally advanced disease, mammography can help in initial staging and follow-up to determine the effects of therapy. Classically, inflammatory breast cancer does not present with a discrete physical or radiographic mass. Rather, the breast is diffusely thickened and the overlying skin is edematous and erythematous (Fig. 4.21). The associated mammogram will reflect these changes, with thickened skin and a diffuse increase in breast parenchemal density. Serial mammograms can complement physical measurements in assessing the response to systemic therapy, which is frequently given before surgery, and/or radiotherapy as so-called "proto"-adjuvant therapy (Fig. 4.22).

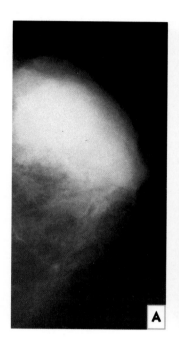
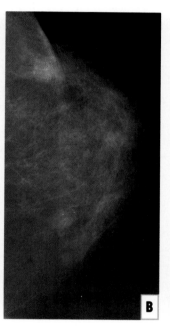
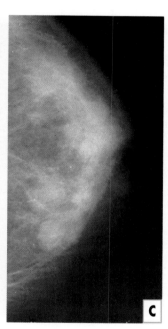

Figure 4.22 Stage IIIB (T4N0) breast cancer. A 45-year-old woman presented with a very large (10-cm) primary tumor. There was an inflammatory component, but a distinct underlying mass was palpable and quite easily detected on the mammogram (A). (B) After chemotherapy and radiotherapy the mass completely disappeared, replaced only by the distortion artifact left by the biopsy. Three months later the tumor recurred within the same breast. (C) The mammogram demonstrates multiple nodular tumor masses and skin thickening. (From Hayes, 1991.)

SUGGESTED READING

Andersson I, Aspegren K, Janzon L, et al. (1988) Mammographic screening and mortality from breast cancer: the Malmö mammographic screening trial. Br Med J 297:943–948.

Baker LH. (1982) Breast cancer detection demonstration project: five year summary report. CA 32:194–225.

Chu KC, Smart CR, Tarone RE. (1988) Analysis of breast cancer mortality and stage distribution by age for the Health Insurance Plan clinical trial. J Natl Cancer Inst 80:1125–1132.

Ciatto S, Cataliotti L, Distante V. (1989) Nonpalpable lesions detected with mammography: review of 512 consecutive cases. Radiology 165:99–102.

Dowlatshahi K, Gent HJ, Schmidt R, et al. (1989) Nonpalpable breast tumors: diagnosis with stereotactic localization and fine-needle aspiration. Radiology 170:427–433.

Eddy DM, Hasselblad V, McGivney W, Hendee W. (1988) The value of mammography screening in women under age 50 years. JAMA 259:1512–1519.

Feig SA. (1984) Radiation risks from mammography: is it clinically significant? AJR 143:469–475.

Hall FM, Storella JM, Silverstone DZ, et al. (1988) Nonpalpable breast lesions: recommendations for biopsy based on suspicion of carcinoma at mammography. Radiology 167:353–358.

Hayes DF. (1991) Breast cancer. In: Skarin AT, ed. *Atlas of Diagnostic Oncology*. New York: Gower Medical Publishing.

Hermann G, Janus C, Schwartz IS, et al. (1987) Nonpalpable breast lesion: accuracy of prebiopsy diagnosis. *Radiology* 165:323–326.

Kopans DB. (1984) "Early" breast cancer detection using technique other than mammography. *AJR* 143:465–488.

Kopans DB. (1989) Fine-needle aspiration of clinically occult breast lesions. *Radiology* 170:313–314.

Kopans DB, Lindfors KK, McCarthy KA, et al. (1985) Spring hookwire breast lesion localizer: use with rigid-compression mammographic systems. *Radiology* 157:537–538.

Kopans DB, Meyer JE, Lindfors KK. (1985) Whole breast ultrasound imaging—four year follow-up. *Radiology* 157:505.

Meyer JE, Kopans DB, Stomper PC, et al. (1984) Occult breast abnormalities: percutaneous preoperative needle localization. *Radiology* 150:335.

Parker SH, Lovin JD, Jobe WE, Luethke JM, et al. (1990) Stereotactic breast biopsy with a biopsy gun. *Radiology* 176:741–747.

Roberts MM, Alexander FE, Anderson TJ, et al. (1990) Edinburgh trial of screening for breast cancer: mortality at seven years [see comments]. *Lancet* 335:241–246.

Sickles EA. (1980) Further experience with microfocal spot magnification mammography in the assessment of clustered breast microcalcifications. *Radiology* 137:9–14.

Sickles EA. (1989) Breast masses: mammographic evaluation. *Radiology* 173:297–303.

Sickles EA. (1991) Periodic mammographic follow-up of probably benign lesions: results in 3,184 consecutive cases. *Radiology* 179:463–468.

Stomper PC. (1992) *Cancer Imaging Manual*. Philadelphia: J.B. Lippincott (in press).

Stomper PC, Connolly JL. (1992) Mammographic features predicting an extensive intraductal component in early stage infiltrating ductal carcinoma. *AJR* 158:269–272.

Stomper PC, Gelman RS. (1989) Mammography in symptomatic and asymptomatic patients. In: Henderson IC, ed. *Hematology/Oncology Clinics of North America*. Philadelphia: W.B. Saunders, 3:611–640.

Stomper PC, Connolly JL, Meyer JE, Harris JR. (1989) Clinically occult ductal carcinoma in situ detected with mammography: analysis of 100 cases with radiologic-pathologic correlation. *Radiology* 172:235–241.

Stomper PC, Davis SP, Meyer JE. (1988) Clinically occult noncalcified breast cancer: serial radiologic-pathologic correlation in 27 cases. *Radiology* 169:621–626.

Stomper PC, Davis SP, Sonnenfeld MR, et al. (1988) Efficiency of specimen radiography of clinically occult noncalcified breast lesions. *AJR* 151:43–47.

Stomper PC, Kopans DB, Sadowsky NL, et al. (1988) Is mammography painful? A multicenter patient survey. *Arch Intern Med* 148:521–524.

Stomper PC, Recht A, Berenberg AL, et al. (1987) Mammographic detection of recurrent cancer in the irradiated breast. *AJR* 148:39–43.

Tabar L, Gad A, Holmberg L, et al. (1985) Reduction in mortality from breast cancer after mass screening with mammography. *Lancet* 2:829–832.

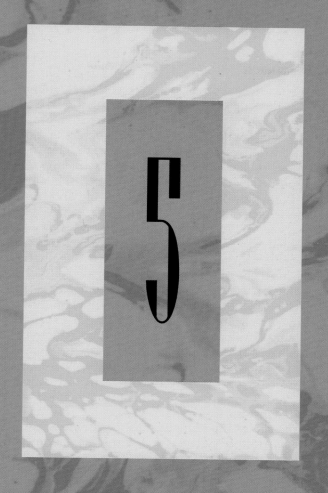

Breast Cancer Surgery

T. J. Eberlein

DIAGNOSIS
History and Physical Examination

As with any new patient, a careful history and physical examination are mandatory in evaluating a patient with a breast cancer. The history should include the patient's personal history as well as her family history of breast cancer (with special attention to maternal first-degree relatives). A meticulous review of other past breast concerns, as well as past medical problems, will assist in planning the patient's therapy, including the type of surgical procedure and the type of anesthetic to be used.

The physical examination is usually done with the patient supine but can be performed with the patient seated with her arms raised over her head (Fig. 5.1). Correlation of a specific area of concern with a mammogram is particularly helpful (see Chapter 4). An important point to emphasize is that, especially in postmenopausal women, pathologic physical evaluation of a palpable mass, even in the event of a negative mammogram, is usually required for a definitive diagnosis.

Biopsy

The technique chosen for biopsy depends on several factors (Fig. 5.2). These include the size of the lesion, whether or not it is palpable, and whether or not it is suspicious for malignancy. The goal of the biopsy (e.g.,

a needle biopsy to document stage III disease or excision of a small but easily palpable stage I cancer), as well as the experience and training of the physician performing the procedure, are also considered in making a choice of biopsy techniques.

Although aspiration is fast and can be done in the office, it provides limited cytologic information (Fig. 5.3). Incisional biopsies (Fig. 5.4A) are more commonly performed. They also can be performed in the outpatient setting and can provide immediate and reliable preliminary pathologic information (see Fig. 5.2). This type of biopsy, however, requires re-excision for definitive treatment. Excisional biopsies (Fig. 5.4A), on the other hand, are also done in the outpatient setting, but they provide additional cytologic information regarding the tumor margins. This type of biopsy, however, may still underestimate the true extent of the tumor margins. An excisional biopsy should be carefully planned, as it may potentially jeopardize definitive treatment with a breast-conserving approach. If excisional therapy is performed and an extensive in situ component of tumor is not seen, radiation therapy is still recommended as primary treatment even when microscopic infiltrating tumor is present at the margins. If extensive in situ disease is present or the margins are macroscopically positive, re-excision or mastectomy is recommended (see below).

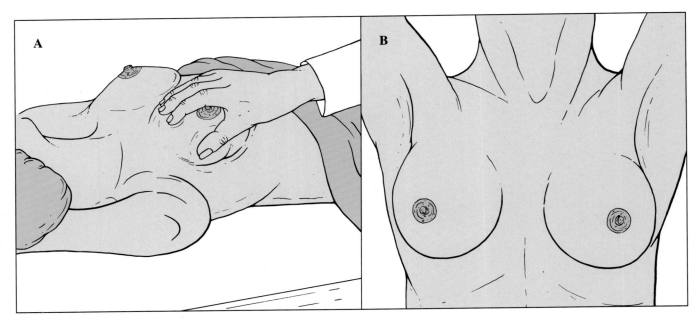

Figure 5.1 Patients with breast masses are most easily examined in the supine position (A), but dimpling and retraction are best seen when the patient is sitting with her arms raised above her head (B).

Figure 5.2 Breast Biopsy Techniques

Type	Advantages	Disadvantages
Aspiration/needle biopsy	Fast; efficient Can be performed in office Local or without anesthesia	Inaccurate or inadequate sample Dependent on experience of pathologist Difficult or unable to evaluate in situ disease ER/PR not available
Incisional biopsy	Relatively fast; frozen section possible ER/PR flow studies obtainable Extent of in situ disease evaluable	Surgical procedure; may understate extent of in situ disease Will require additional surgical procedure to treat
Excisional biopsy	Same as incisional biopsy More complete evaluation of in situ disease Can evaluate margins of excision	Larger procedure May still underestimate true extent of tumor requiring re-excision May make further conservative treatment more difficult
Needle-directed excisional biopsy	Used for nonpalpable abnormalities	Dependent upon skill of radiologist Done in operating room if needed May underestimate extent of tumor May require re-excision
Stereotactic breast biopsy	Accurate image guidance Cost efficient Accurate histology Not done in operating room	Requires special mammography equipment Limited sample size ER/PR may not be available May underestimate in situ disease

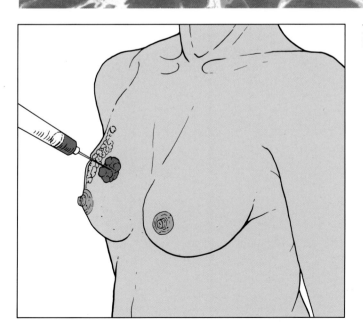

Figure 5.3 A patient undergoing needle aspiration. The mass is fixed with the examiner's hand and a 21-gauge needle is used.

Needle-directed biopsies are used for nonpalpable lesions. Although they require an outpatient procedure room, they can usually be performed without anesthesia or with anesthesia on standby (Fig. 5.5). Stereotactic breast biopsies require special mammographic equipment. This technology is new and therefore unproven. It involves a core biopsy with a 14-gauge needle. This type of biopsy should provide accurate histology, including estrogen receptor (ER) and progesterone receptor (PR) status by ERICA, and also can be done in the outpatient setting.

PRIMARY THERAPY

Conservative Treatment

Several randomized clinical trials recently conducted to compare the outcome of conservative surgery plus radiation with that of mastectomy alone have shown an equivalent rate of survival. However, several caveats

have been raised: the tumors were relatively small and the margins were negative. For example, the NSABP B-06 trial limited tumor to ≤4 cm. The Milan trial studied patients with T1N0 lesions only. The intent of breast-conserving therapy is to preserve satisfactory cosmetics. Therefore, certain surgical techniques have been developed that minimize disruption of normal breast and skin. General principles of breast-conserving surgery are listed in Figure 5.6.

As with mastectomy (see below), the obvious risks of conservative surgery include infection, bleeding, scarring or deformity of the breast, and possible injury to the thoracodorsal or long thoracic nerve, as well as possible edema of the arm after node dissection. Breast deformity can be minimized by using circumferential-type incisions in the upper half of the breast (Fig. 5.7) and radial incision in the lower half of the breast (see Fig. 5.7). Cosmesis is also aided by performing the dissection excision at a tangent to the skin so that the

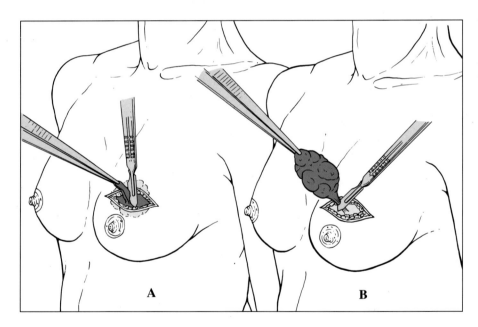

Figure 5.4 (A) An incisional biopsy makes a definitive diagnosis. (B) Excisional biopsies, although diagnostic, can also be therapeutic by eliminating the need for further breast surgery when radiation therapy is performed.

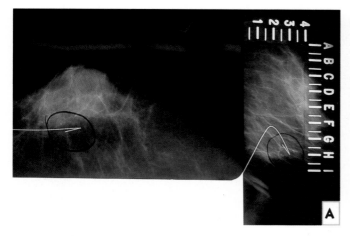

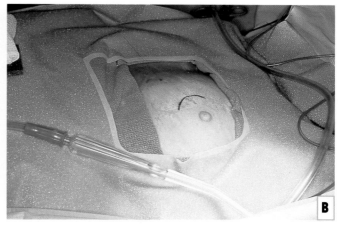

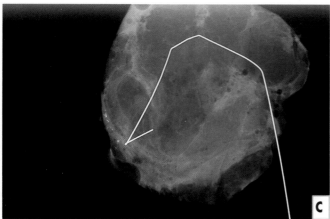

Figure 5.5 (A) Mammograms of postmenopausal woman with microcalcifications in the left breast. (B) The incision is placed as central in the breast and as close to the actual abnormality as possible. (C) Specimen mammograms are utilized to determine whether the microcalifications have been excised.

Figure 5.6 Breast-conserving surgery

Keep incision central

Limit volume of breast tissue removed

Limit amount of skin excised

Ensure good hemostasis

Avoid drains in breast

Separate breast and axillary incisions

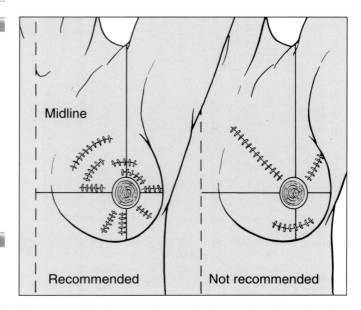

Figure 5.7 Cosmesis is best maintained using circular incisions in the upper half of the breast and radial incisions in the lower half of the breast.

cavity will close as two flaps with a minimum of suturing (Fig. 5.8). The volume of breast excised and the amount of skin removed should be as small as possible. Care should also be taken to ensure meticulous hemostasis so that drains will be unnecessary. Separate incisions for the breast and axillary surgeries are preferred.

One factor associated with a higher risk of recurrence in the breast is the presence of extensive intraductal component (EIC) within and surrounding the invasive elements of the tumor. An important feature of this so-called extensive intraductal component is that intraductal carcinoma not only is prominently present within the tumor but is also present in the grossly normal surrounding tissue. Although the presence of EIC does not appear to predict distant recurrence or death from breast cancer, most physicians feel that when cancer recurs in an irradiated breast, mastectomy is the treatment of choice (since the normal breast tissue cannot tolerate more radiation than is used in the original primary therapy). The risk of breast recurrence in women who have EIC may be as high as 25 percent after five years of followup. When EIC is present (see

Chapter 9), larger resections achieve smaller recurrence rates. When the tumor is EIC negative, simple excision is adequate. Therefore, when a patient has a T_0 or T_1 tumor, she should undergo gross excision with inked margins (see Chapter 6). When the tumor is EIC negative, the patient's primary treatment may be completed with radiation therapy. If the tumor is EIC positive, the patient has a choice of mastectomy or wide excision with inked margins. If the margins of the wide excision are negative, the patient may be treated with radiation. Alternatively, if the margins of the wide excision are positive, mastectomy should be performed (Fig. 5.9). Patients with T_2 tumors should undergo incisional biopsy. If this biopsy is EIC positive, gross excision with inked margins under general anesthesia is indicated, followed by radiation therapy. If the biopsy reveals an EIC positive tumor, the patient should undergo mastectomy or wide excision with inked margins. Patients with negative margins are candidates for breast conservation with radiation therapy, but those with positive margins will require a mastectomy (Fig. 5.10). Unfavorable results of conservative surgery stemming from poor

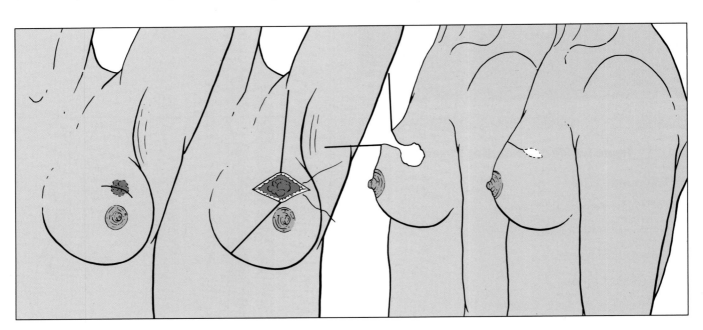

Figure 5.8 In performing breast-conserving surgery, one should strive to excise tissue at a tangent to the skin, thereby resulting in a "flap" closure that minimizes the number of sutures used to close the cavity and obliterate the dead space.

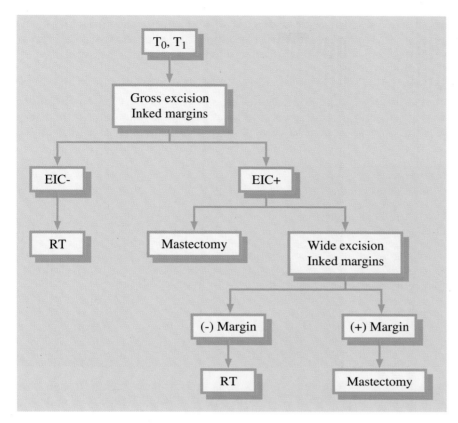

Figure 5.9 Algorithm for treatment of T_0, T_1 breast cancer.

Figure 5.10 Algorithm for treatment of T_2 breast cancer.

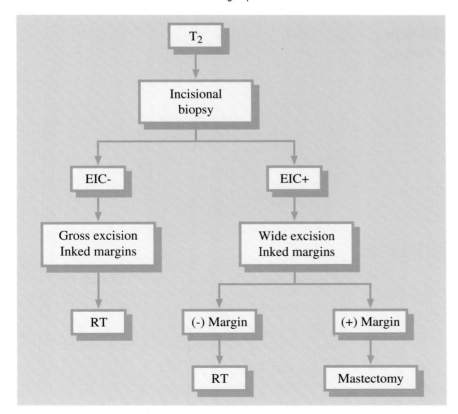

surgical techniques are shown in Figure 5.11. The desired results are shown in Figure 5.12.

In summary, breast-conserving surgery requires careful evaluation of the prebiopsy mammogram, the presence or absence of EIC, and the location of the tumor with respect to the margins of excision. Postbiopsy mammograms with magnification views may be necessary to evaluate residual abnormalities. It is important to remember that ductal carcinoma in situ (DCIS) tracks toward the nipple and the frozen section report must be distrusted when re-excision is performed.

Mastectomy

The indications for mastectomy are listed in Figure 5.13. Figure 5.14 also depicts an indication for mastectomy. Whereas some indications, such as multifocal or

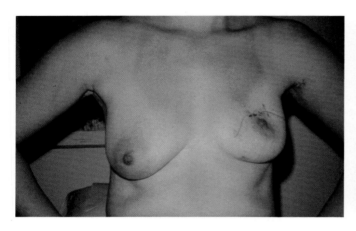

Figure 5.11 Poor results resulting from removal of excessive skin and breast tissue, leading to extensive volume loss in the breast and severe displacement of the nipple.

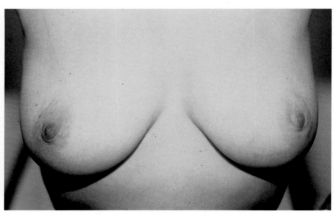

Figure 5.12 The desired cosmetic result for conservative surgery/radiation therapy. Which side had the cancer?

Figure 5.13 Indications for Mastectomy (Relative Contraindications for Breast-Conserving Therapy)

Patient preference

Diffuse or multifocal disease

Medical contraindication to radiotherapy

Pregnancy

Anticipated poor cosmetic result

Quality of radiation therapy

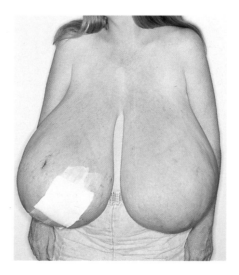

Figure 5.14 A 26-week pregnant woman with massive breast hypertrophy that caused bilateral ulceration of the skin and bleeding. Thirty-four pounds of breast tissue were removed during bilateral mastectomies.

diffuse disease and pregnancy, are objective, some other indications, such as preference, anticipated poor cosmetic result with conservative surgery, and quality and/or availability of radiation therapy, are clearly subjective. In general, the nipple and areola, as well as the old biopsy incision, should be widely excised (Fig. 5.15). En block resection of the axilla (Fig. 5.16) is preferred, as this technique preserves the intercostal brachial nerve, the thoracodorsal vessels and nerve,

and the long thoracic nerve (Fig. 5.17). Closure is accomplished with a subcuticular suture (Fig. 5.18). Depending on the clinical situation, a level I or level II axillary dissection can be performed (Fig. 5.19). For example, a level I dissection or sampling might be sufficient in the case of extensive DCIS without invasion or for the elderly patient. Total axillary or level III dissection is usually not done in breast cancer, since it neither permits more adequate staging nor prevents

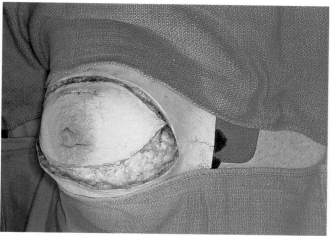

Figure 5.15 Mastectomy incision including the old biopsy scar as well as the nipple and areola.

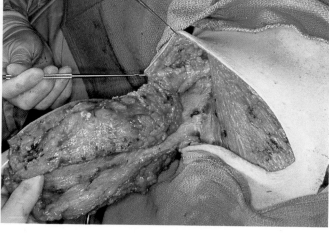

Figure 5.16 Axillary dissection is done en bloc with the breast specimen.

Figure 5.17 Axillary dissection preserves the intercostal brachial nerve, as well as the thoracodorsal vessels and nerve and the long thoracic nerve.

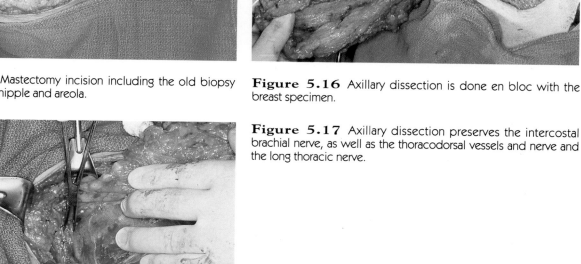

axillary recurrence. It will certainly, however, increase the risk of postoperative arm edema. This complication can be devastating and is more common when level III dissection is coupled with axillary radiation therapy (Fig. 5.20).

Patients who require mastectomy are also encouraged to undergo immediate reconstruction. Although this lengthens the time of surgery and hospital stay, there are few situations in medicine that uniformly produce such overwhelming patient satisfaction. Two general procedures for reconstruction are performed. One involves the use of artificial implants or expanders (Fig. 5.21), and the other utilizes the patient's own tissue. Reconstruction can be done with little morbidity (Fig. 5.22).

A patient with bilateral mastectomies is shown in Figure 5.23A. The same patient is shown after bilateral silicone implants in Figure 5.23B and C. These implants are inserted under the pectoralis major muscle as shown in Figure 5.24. When the mastectomy leaves insufficient skin to place a permanent implant, a second type of reconstruction is performed. A tissue expander is placed under the pectoralis major muscle (Fig. 5.25A–D), and after a sufficient pocket has been created with the expander a second surgical procedure is performed to replace the tissue expander with a permanent silicone implant (Fig. 5.25E). Implants/expanders are advantageous because they are relatively quick surgical procedures that produce good cosmetic results, especially in small breasts. Disadvantages include infection, which

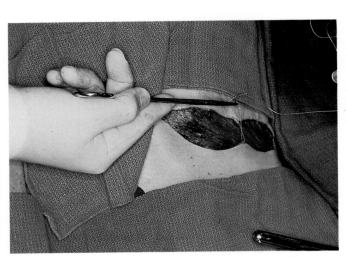

Figure 5.18 Closure of a mastectomy wound without reconstruction is accomplished with subcuticular or plastic closure.

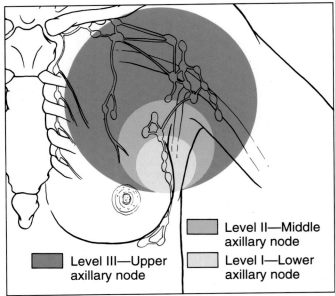

Level II—Middle axillary node

Level III—Upper axillary node

Level I—Lower axillary node

Figure 5.19 Extent of axillary dissection. Level I sampling includes the nodes around the axillary tail of the breast. Level II removes the nodes up to the axillary vein. Level III removes all the nodes, including nodes above the axillary vein and underneath the pectoralis major. (Adapted from Hayes, 1991.)

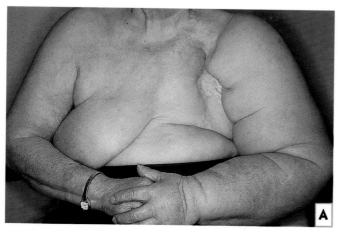

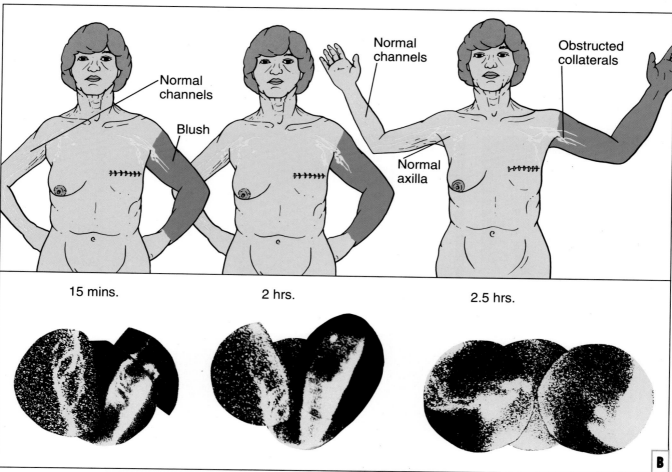

Figure 5.20 (A) A 64-year-old patient with significant arm edema after a radical mastectomy, full axillary dissection, and postoperative chest wall and axillary radiotherapy. The patient's left arm is immensely swollen in contrast to her unaffected, normal right arm. After subcutaneous injection of radionuclide into the dorsa of each hand, scintograms were obtained (B). In the anterior views at 15 minutes and two hours, flow can easily be seen in nor- mal channels in the right arm. However, only a "blush" can be seen in the left because the normal lymph channels are occluded, and the radionuclide is present only in small collateral channels that do not communicate with distal vessels. In the view of the thorax at 2.5 hours, flow can be seen on the right side in normal channels leading to axillary lymph nodes. On contrast, radionuclide has accumulated in the lower arm and is absent in the left axilla.

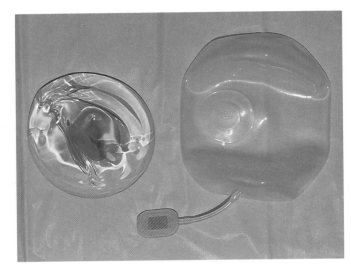

Figure 5.21 Silicone implant (*left*) and tissue expander inflated with saline (*right*).

Figure 5.22 Incidence of Complications with TRAM Flap Versus Tissue Expander/Implant Reconstruction

Type of Complication	Incidence (%)	Tissue Expander/ Implant
Infection	1.1	0.7
Hematoma	1.1	3.1
Weak abdominal fascia	3.3	0
Chest flap necrosis	3.3	3.9
Flap necrosis <20%	6.7	0
Cardiac	1.1	0

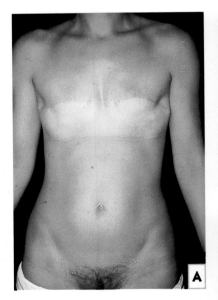

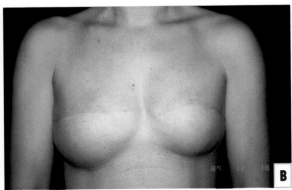

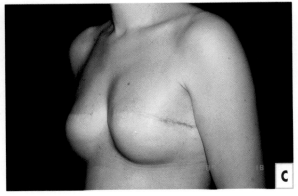

Figure 5.23 (A) A patient with bilateral mastectomies. (B,C) Frontal and side views of same patient after bilateral silicone implants.

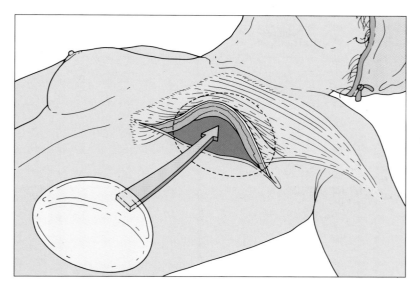

Figure 5.24 A submuscular pocket under the pectoralis major is created to receive the silicone implant. (From Vasconez, LeJour, and Gamboa-Bobadilla, 1991.)

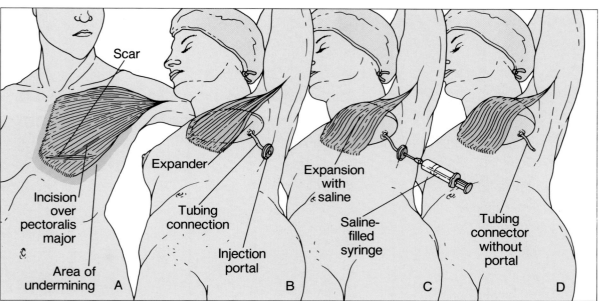

Scar

Expander

Expansion with saline

Tubing connector without portal

Incision over pectoralis major

Tubing connection

Saline-filled syringe

Injection portal

Area of undermining

A B C D

Figure 5.25 (A–D) A tissue expander is placed under the pectoralis major muscle and expanded until a sufficient sized pocket has been created. (E) The expander is then usually replaced with a permanent implant. (From Vasconez, LeJour, and Gamboa-Bobadilla, 1991.)

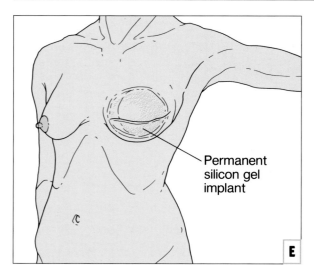

Permanent silicon gel implant

E

Breast Cancer Surgery

requires removal of the implant, encapsulation or hardening of the scar around the implant, leaking of silicone, and, in patients treated with expanders, the need for an additional surgical procedure.

An increasingly attractive alternative to implants is the use of the patient's own tissue. These musculocutaneous flaps are based on rotation of an individual artery and vein to maintain the blood supply and the viability of their tissue. An example of one of these flaps is the latissimus dorsi myocutaneous flap (Fig. 5.26). This flap is usually based on the thoracodorsal artery and vein and is often used in combination with an implant as the latissimus dorsi muscle is not large enough in most women. The resultant scar on the back is well hidden (Fig. 5.27A). This flap can provide an excellent overall cosmetic result (Fig. 5.27B and C).

An alternative myocutaneous flap is the transverse rectus abdominus muscle (TRAM) flap. This procedure

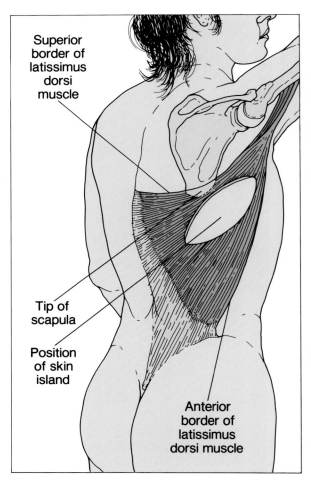

Figure 5.26 The latissimus dorsi myocutaneous flap is based on the thoracodorsal artery and vein. This flap is rotated from the back and becomes the breast mound. (From Vasconez, LeJour, and Gamboa-Bobadilla, 1991.)

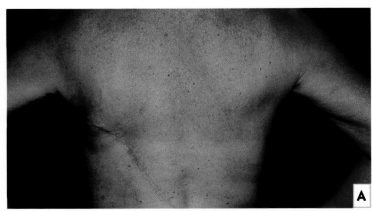

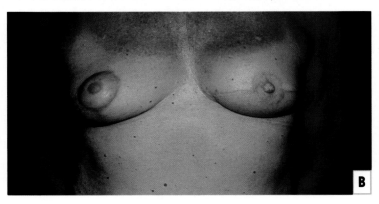

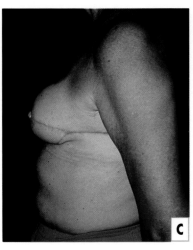

Figure 5.27 (A) The resultant scar from harvesting a latissimus flap. (B,C) The resulting cosmetic effect after reconstruction with a latissimus flap.

is particularly advantageous in large-breasted women when additional tissue coverage is needed. Obviously, extensive prior abdominal surgery contraindicates such a procedure. The TRAM flap is based on the superior epigastric artery and vein (Fig. 5.28), can be used for reconstructing the contralateral breast as well as the ipsilateral breast, and results in a low bikini scar (Fig. 5.29A–C). This type of reconstruction gives a superb appearance and a natural feel to the reconstructed breast (Fig. 5.30A and B). Free flaps can also be used for reconstruction through microsurgical techniques, for example, with gluteal (buttock) muscle. The advantages of tissue flaps for mastectomy reconstruction include excellent cosmetic results and more natural breast contours and feel.

The disadvantages of the tissue flap procedure include more complex and lengthy surgical procedures, longer hospitalizations, and occasionally minor tissue necrosis and abdominal hernia, which occur in approximately 1 percent of patients after TRAM flaps. In a prospective series of over 200 mastectomies and immediate reconstructions, complications were minimal yet patient satisfaction was very high.

Patients overwhelmingly state that they would consent again to breast reconstruction and would not hesitate to recommend the surgery to others. Therefore, in the patient who requires or desires mastectomy as treatment for breast cancer, a cosmetically acceptable alternative to mastectomy alone is now available.

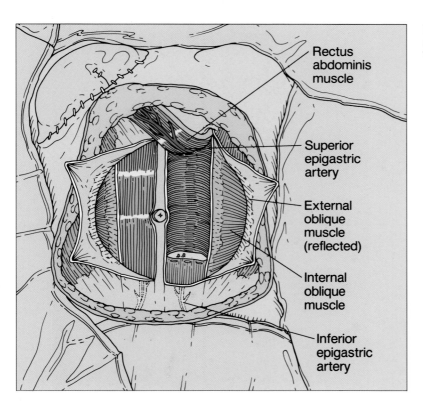

Rectus abdominis muscle

Superior epigastric artery

External oblique muscle (reflected)

Internal oblique muscle

Inferior epigastric artery

Figure 5.28 The anatomy of a transverse rectus abdominal myocutaneous (TRAM) flap. (From Vasconez, LeJour, and Gamboa-Bobadilla, 1991.)

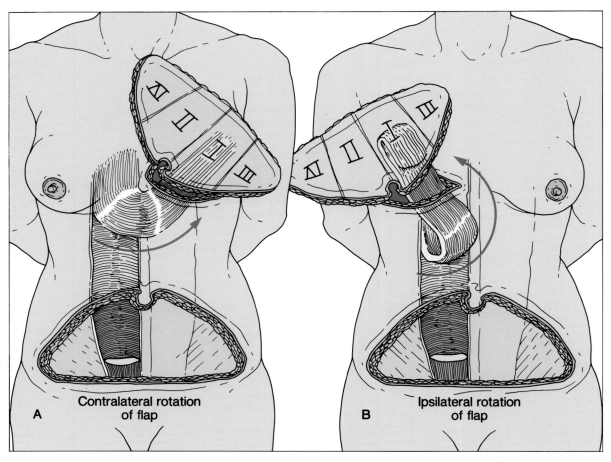

Contralateral rotation of flap

A

Ipsilateral rotation of flap

B

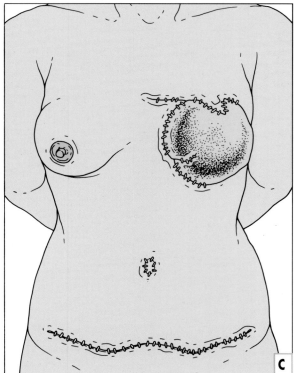

C

Figure 5.29 A TRAM flap can be used to reconstruct (A) the contralateral breast and (B) the ipsilateral breast. (C) A low bikini-type incision. (From Vasconez, LeJour, and Gamboa-Bobadilla, 1991.)

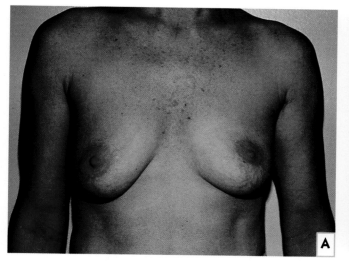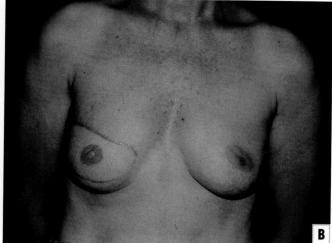

Figure 5.30 (A) Before mastectomy. (B) The same patient after mastectomy and TRAM flap reconstruction.

SUGGESTED READING

Boyages J, Recht A, Connolly JP, et al. (1990) Early breast cancer: predictors of breast recurrence for breast cancer patients treated with conservative surgery and radiation therapy. *Radiother Oncol* 19:29–41.

Eberlein TJ, Connolly JL, Schnitt SJ, Recht A, Osteen RT, Harris JR. (1990) Predictors of local recurrence following surgery and radiation therapy: the influence of tumor size. *Arch Surg* 125:771–777.

Fisher B, Redmond C, Poisson R, et al. (1989) Eight-year results of a randomized clinical trial comparing total mastectomy and lumpectomy with or without irradiation in the treatment of breast cancer. *N Engl J Med* 320:822–828.

Harris JR, Recht A. (1991) Conservative surgery and radiotherapy. In: Harris JR, Hellman S, Henderson IC, Kinne D, eds. *Breast Diseases*. Philadelphia: JB Lippincott, 389.

Hayes DF. (1991) Breast cancer. In: Skarin AT, ed. *Atlas of Diagnostic Oncology*. New York: Gower Medical Publishing.

Parker SH, Lovin JD, Jobe WE, et al. (1990) Steretactic breast biopsy with a biopsy gun. *Radiology* 176:741–747.

Vasconez LO, LeJour H, Gamboa-Bobadilla M. (1991) *Atlas of Breast Reconstruction*. New York: Gower Medical Publishing.

Veronesi U. (1987) Rationale and indications for limited surgery in breast cancer: current data. *World J Surg* 11:493–498.

Vicini FA, Eberlein TJ, Connolly JL, et al. (1991) Extent of resection for patients with stage I-II breast cancer treated with conservative surgery (CS) and radiotherapy (RT). *Ann Surg* 214:200–205.

6

Processing of Breast Biopsies

Stuart J. Schnitt

This permits confirmation that the mammographically suspicious lesion has been removed and also directs the pathologist to the location within the specimen of the area of interest (Fig. 6.3).

SPECIAL STUDIES

A variety of special studies can be used to supplement the routine histologic evaluation of breast tumors. These include estrogen and progesterone receptor analyses, electron microscopy, flow cytometry and other methods to assess DNA content and proliferative rate, immunohistochemical studies for a broad range of antigens, methods to analyze oncogene amplification and expression, and morphometric analysis. Consideration of each of these methods is beyond the scope of this atlas. However, a discussion of estrogen and progesterone receptor analysis is in order, since assays for these receptors are the most widely applied and clinically useful of these supplemental techniques.

Measurement of estrogen and progesterone receptor content provides useful clinical information regarding both the likelihood of response to endocrine therapy and the prognosis. Several different methods are presently in use to determine the estrogen and progesterone receptor content of breast tumors. These methods can be broadly divided into two categories: biochemical assays and immunohistochemical assays. The most widely used biochemical assay is the dextran-coat-ed charcoal (DCC) method. In this assay, breast tumor cytosol is incubated with radioactive hormone. DCC is added to this mixture and serves to adsorb unbound hormone. Centrifugation is used to separate the heavier DCC-bound hormone from the receptor-bound hormone, which is present in the supernatant. The quantity of receptor-bound hormone is determined by analyzing an aliquot of the supernatant in a scintillation counter. The most widely used immunohistochemical assays employ incubation of cytologic or histologic preparations of the tumor with monoclonal antibodies to the receptor protein. The antibody–receptor complex can then be visualized using an immunoenzyme detection system (e.g., immunoalkaline phosphatase or immunoperoxidase) (Fig. 6.4). The reagents for the immunohistochemical analysis for both estrogen receptor and progesterone receptor are commercially available in kit form [known as the estrogen receptor immunocytochemical assay (ERICA) and the progesterone receptor immunocytochemical assay (PgRICA), respectively]. Biochemical and immunohistochemical assays each have their advantages and disadvantages, as shown in Figure 6.5. At present, when a sufficient amount of tissue is available, the biochemical method is the assay of choice. However, the immunohistochemical method is extremely useful for evaluation of hormone receptors in small tissue specimens and in cytologic preparations (e.g., from effusions or fine-needle aspirates).

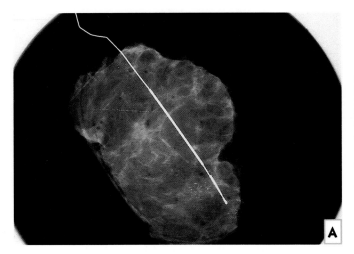
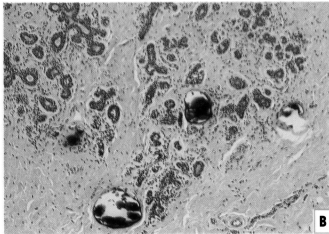

Figure 6.3 (A) Specimen radiograph with localization wire in situ demonstrating microcalcifications near the end of the wire; (B) in this case, calcifications were microscopically observed only in normal lobules.

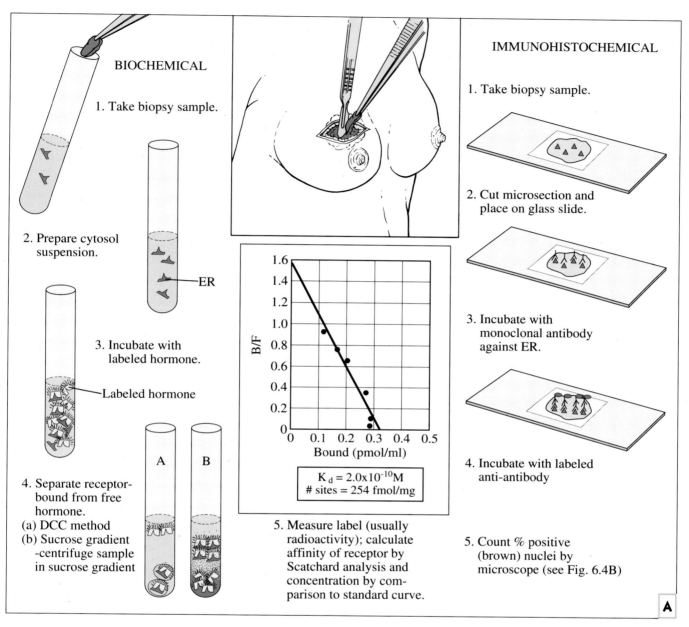

BIOCHEMICAL

1. Take biopsy sample.

2. Prepare cytosol suspension.

— ER

3. Incubate with labeled hormone.

— Labeled hormone

4. Separate receptor-bound from free hormone.
(a) DCC method
(b) Sucrose gradient -centrifuge sample in sucrose gradient

$K_d = 2.0 \times 10^{-10} M$
sites = 254 fmol/mg

5. Measure label (usually radioactivity); calculate affinity of receptor by Scatchard analysis and concentration by comparison to standard curve.

IMMUNOHISTOCHEMICAL

1. Take biopsy sample.

2. Cut microsection and place on glass slide.

3. Incubate with monoclonal antibody against ER.

4. Incubate with labeled anti-antibody

5. Count % positive (brown) nuclei by microscope (see Fig. 6.4B)

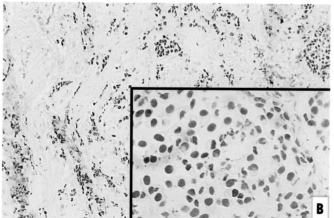

Figure 6.4 (A) Assays for steroid hormone receptors. Scatchard analysis of [³H] estradiol binding to estrogen receptor (ER) in human breast cancer cytosol, determined by the multipoint DDC assay. The calculated binding affinity (K_d) and the quantitative receptor content are shown. (B) Localization of estrogen receptor protein using the estrogen receptor immunocytochemical assay (ERICA). In this frozen section of an infiltrating ductal carcinoma, a brown stain in the nucleus defines the presence of estrogen receptor. Although most cells in this tumor show immunoreactivity, there is heterogeneity in the degree of reactivity among the tumor cells. (From Hayes, 1991.)

Processing of Breast Biopsies

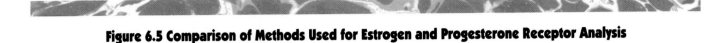

Figure 6.5 Comparison of Methods Used for Estrogen and Progesterone Receptor Analysis

	Biochemical	Immunohistochemical
Minimum amount of tissue required	100 mg	Small number of tumor cells
Type of preparation used in assay	Tissue homogenates (cytosol)	Tissue sections, cytologic preparations
Direct visualization of cells analyzed	No	Yes
Assessment of tumor cell heterogeneity	No	Yes
Nature of receptor analyzed	Free (unbound) only	Free or bound
Radioactive label required	Yes	No
Type of results	Objective, quantitative	Subjective, semiquantitative

SUGGESTED READING

Connolly JL, Schnitt SJ. (1988) Evaluation of breast biopsy specimens in patients considered for treatment by conservative surgery and radiation therapy for early breast cancer. *Pathol Annu* 23[Part I]:1–23.

Hayes DF. (1991) Breast cancer. In: Skarin AT, ed. *Atlas of Diagnostic Onology*. New York: Gower Medical Publishing, 6.1–6.31.

Kline TS, Kline IK. (1989) *Guides to Clinical Aspiration Biopsy—Breast*. New York: Igak Gu-Shoin.

Osborne CK. (1991) Receptors. In: Harris JR, Hellman S, Henderson IC, Kinne DW, eds. *Breast Diseases*, 2nd ed. Philadelphia: JB Lippincott, 301–325.

Owings D, Hann L, Schnitt SJ. (1990) How thoroughly should needle localization breast biopsies be sampled for microscopic examination? A prospective mammographic–pathologic correlative study. *Am J Surg Pathol* 14:578–583.

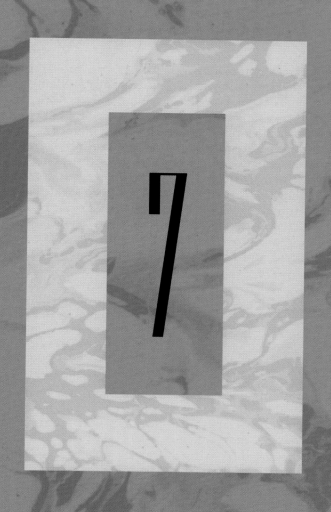

Benign Breast Disorders

Stuart J. Schnitt

Benign breast disorders constitute a heterogeneous group of lesions which, clinically and radiographically, span the entire spectrum of breast abnormalities. The importance of these lesions is twofold. First, some benign breast lesions present as palpable and/or radiographic masses and must therefore be distinguished from cancers. Second, recent studies have indicated that histologic categorization of benign breast lesions provides useful information regarding the patient's risk of subsequently developing breast cancer.

Benign breast lesions can be broadly divided into two groups: fibrocystic changes, a wastebasket term encompassing a variety of clinical and histologic changes, and distinct entities.

FIBROCYSTIC CHANGES

Although the terms *fibrocystic changes* or *fibrocystic disease* are frequently used by clinicians and pathologists, they do not represent a distinct entity either clinically or pathologically. Clinically, these terms have been used to describe a condition characterized by palpable masses in the breast that fluctuate during the course of the menstrual cycle and that may be associated with breast tenderness and/or pain. However, most women have such signs and symptoms at some time in their lives, and these palpable lumps in many cases probably represent physiologic alterations rather than pathologic processes. Pathologically, the lesions subsumed under this heading include macroscopic and microscopic cysts, stromal fibrosis, apocrine metaplasia, and a variety of epithelial proliferative lesions. However, autopsy studies have shown that such changes are virtually ubiquitous in female breasts. Therefore, fibrocystic change/fibrocystic disease is neither a clinically nor a pathologically discrete entity.

The use of the term fibrocystic disease would have little importance were it not for the fact that this disorder has been said to increase a patient's risk of developing breast cancer. However, a number of recent studies have clearly shown that all patients with so-called fibrocystic disease are not at the same risk and that, on the basis of the histologic components of fibrocystic disease, patients can be divided into subgroups with different degrees of risk for the development of breast cancer. When this information is combined with other factors such as family history and age, subgroups of patients can be identified who are at substantially greater risk of developing breast cancer than the general population.

A system for histologically categorizing benign breast lesions into distinct subgroups with differing clinical implications has been developed by Dupont and Page (1985), based on the results of a large follow-up study of women with benign breast lesions, and has been endorsed by the College of American Pathologists. This system separates the various components of the fibrocystic complex into three groups, each with a different risk for the development of subsequent breast cancer. This system is presented in Figures 7.1 and 7.2, and the lesions are illustrated in Figures 7.3 through 7.11.

Figure 7.1 Categorization of Benign Breast Lesions Based on Risk of Developing Subsequent Breast Cancer*

No increased risk (nonproliferative lesions)		Slightly increased risk (proliferative lesions without atypia)		Moderately increased risk (atypical hyperplasias)	
Cysts†	(Fig. 7.3)	Moderate or florid hyperplasia	(Fig. 7.7)	Atypical ductal hyperplasia	(Fig. 7.10)
Apocrine metaplasia	(Fig. 7.4)	Intraductal papilloma	(Fig. 7.8)	Atypical lobular hyperplasia	(Fig. 7.11)
Mild hyperplasia	(Fig. 7.5)	Sclerosing adenosis	(Fig. 7.9)		
Fibroadenomas	(Fig. 7.6)				

* Modified from Page (1986) and College of American Pathologists Consensus Statement (1986).
†Some investigators have reported that macroscopic cysts are associated with a slightly increased risk.

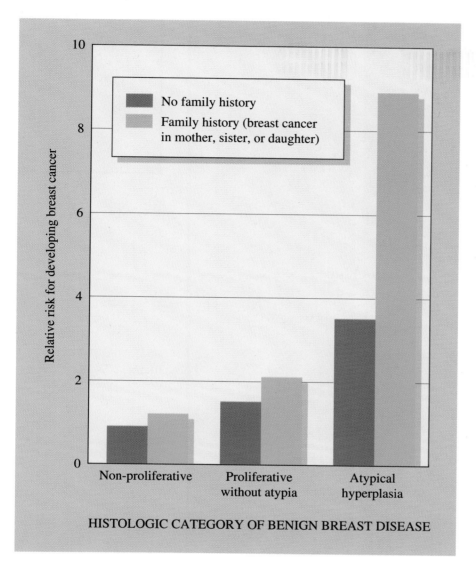

Figure 7.2 Relative risk of breast cancer for women with nonproliferative lesions, proliferative lesions without atypia and atypical hyperplasia, with and without a family history of breast cancer. (Adapted from Dupont and Page, 1985.)

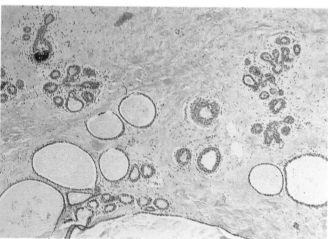

Figure 7.3 Microscopic cysts. Cysts are derived from the terminal duct lobular unit. The epithelium typically consists of two layers: an inner (luminal) epithelial layer and an outer myoepithelial layer. In some cysts, the epithelium becomes attenuated or may be absent. In others the epithelium shows apocrine metaplasia (see Fig. 7.4). Cysts often contain amorphous proteinaceous secretions. (From Hayes, 1991.)

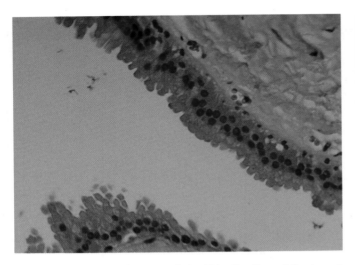

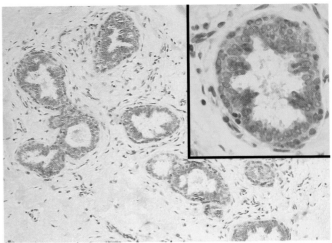

Figure 7.4 Apocrine metaplasia. This alteration of the breast epithelium is characterized by cuboidal to columnar cells which show round nuclei, abundant granular eosinophilic cytoplasm, and "decapitation" secretion.

Figure 7.5 Mild hyperplasia is characterized by an increase in ductal epithelial cells that is more than two but not more than four cells in depth. The epithelial cells do not cross the duct lumen. (From Hayes, 1991.)

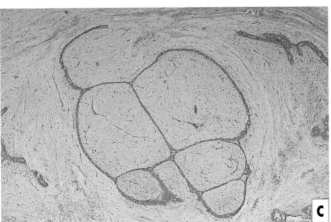

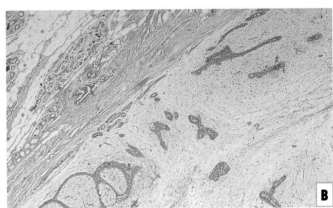

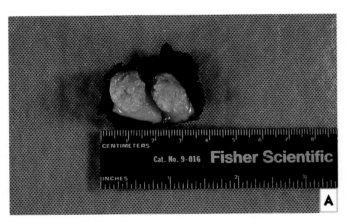

Figure 7.6 Fibroadenoma. (A) Gross photograph of a fibroadenoma. The tumor is well circumscribed and bulges above the cut surface of the specimen. (B,C) Photomicrographs illustrating the histologic features. These lesions most often occur in younger women. They are macroscopically and microscopically well circumscribed and are composed of benign stromal and epithelial elements.

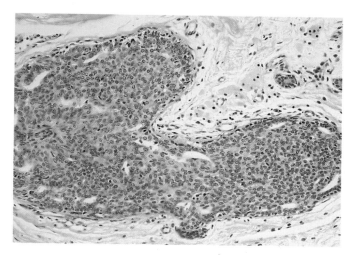

Figure 7.7 Florid hyperplasia. This proliferative lesion is characterized by benign epithelial cells that fill and distend the involved duct. The nuclei vary in shape, size, and orientation. The residual spaces in the duct also vary in size and shape. (From Hayes, 1991.)

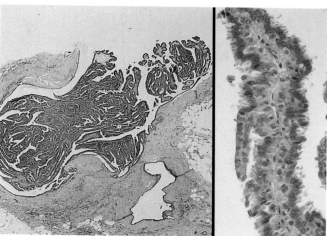

Figure 7.8 Intraductal papilloma. Low-magnification view shows a large duct filled with a papillary lesion. At higher power, the papillae are shown to consist of a central fibrovascular core which is covered by two cell layers, an epithelial layer (closer to the duct lumen) and a myoepithelial layer (lying closer to the core). These lesions usually present with bloody nipple discharge. (From Hayes, 1991.)

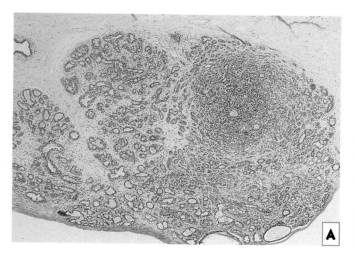

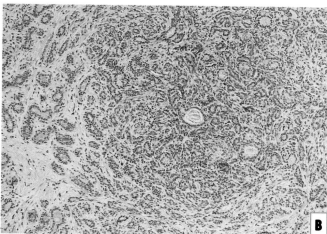

Figure 7.9 Sclerosing adenosis. (A) Low-power view; (B) higher-power view. This lesion consists of a proliferation of glandular structures and stroma in a lobulocentric configuration. These glands may become compressed and distorted by the fibrous stroma, producing a pattern that may mimic infiltrating cancer. Although usually a microscopic finding, sclerosing adenosis may present as a palpable mass ("adenosis tumor"). (From Hayes, 1991.)

SPECIFIC ENTITIES

A variety of benign neoplasms and reactive/inflammatory lesions may present as masses on clinical examination and/or imaging studies and must be distinguished from cancers. The most common benign neoplasm of the female breast is the fibroadenoma (see Fig. 7.6). Intraductal papillomas are also fairly common but more typically present with nipple discharge rather than a palpable mass (see Fig. 7.8). Two of the more frequent reactive/inflammatory lesions are fat necrosis (Fig. 7.12) and mammary duct ectasia (see Fig. 7.13). Less common

lesions that present as masses on either physical examination or radiographic studies include hamartomas (Fig. 7.14), radial scars (Fig. 7.15), and granular cell tumors (Fig. 7.16). It is important to note that some of these benign lesions, particularly fat necrosis, radial scars, and granular cell tumors, can closely mimic carcinomas on clinical, radiographic, and even on macroscopic pathologic examination. Gynecomastia is the most frequent benign abnormality of the male breast (Fig. 7.17). This may be unilateral or bilateral and may present as either a distinct mass or diffuse enlargement of the breast.

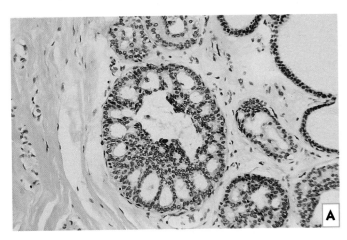 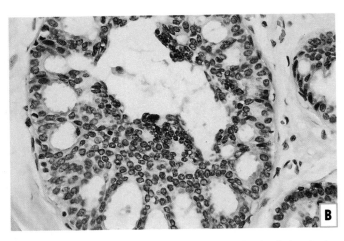

Figure 7.10 Atypical ductal hyperplasia. (A) Low-power view; (B) higher-power view. This epithelial proliferation has some but not all of the features of ductal carcinoma in situ. Near the center of the duct there is a population of relatively round, uniform epithelial cells with regularly placed nuclei. However, these cells comprise only a portion of the lesion. In other areas (e.g., near the periphery of the duct), the epithelial cells maintain their orientation. In addition, although some of the spaces in this proliferation are relatively round and regular, there is still some variation in the size and shape of the spaces. Since this lesion has features intermediate between those of ductal carcinoma in situ and florid hyperplasia, it is designated "atypical ductal hyperplasia."

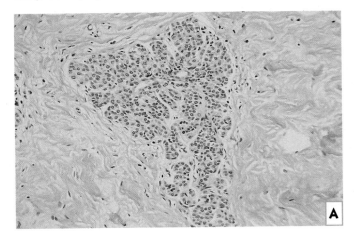 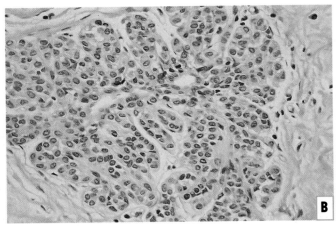

Figure 7.11 Atypical lobular hyperplasia. (A) Low-power view; (B) higher-power view. This lesion is characterized by a proliferation of small, uniform cells in the acini. The cells are dyscohesive, and the involved acini are not distended by this process. Since this proliferation has some but not all, of the features of lobular carcinoma in situ it is classified as "atypical lobular hyperplasia."

TREATMENT EFFECTS

A variety of pathologic changes attributable to radiation therapy and chemotherapy have been observed in benign breast tissue. Patients with early stage breast cancer who have been treated by local excision followed by radiation therapy occasionally develop areas of fat necrosis in the vicinity of the primary tumor. These lesions must be surgically excised to distinguish them from recurrent neoplasm. Pathologically, these lesions are identical to fat necrosis occurring in the nonirradiated breast (see Fig. 7.12). Irradiated normal breast tissue characteristically shows atypical epithelial cells in the terminal duct lobular unit, associated with variable degrees of lobular atrophy (Fig. 7.18). Similar changes have been observed in nontumorous breast tissue after chemotherapy.

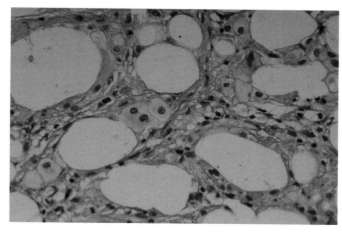

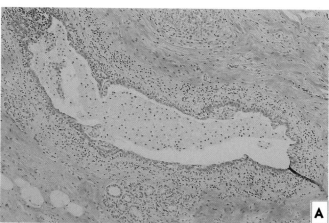

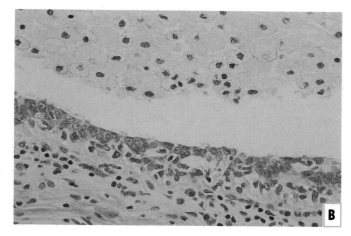

Figure 7.12 Fat necrosis. The adipose tissue of the breast is infiltrated with histiocytes that contain foamy cytoplasm. A history of breast trauma is elicited in less than 50 percent of patients with fat necrosis.

Figure 7.13 Duct ectasia. (A) Low-power view shows an ectatic duct with inspissated secretion and intraluminal histiocytes. There is mild periductal chronic inflammation. (B) Higher magnification shows histiocytes within the duct lumen and mononuclear inflammatory cells around the duct. This disorder involves the extralobular ducts. In the early stages there is stasis of secretions within the duct lumen (often accompanied by histiocytes) and periductal chronic inflammation. In the later stages periductal fibrosis occurs, and this phenomenon may produce nipple retraction.

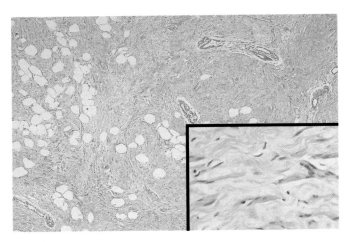

Figure 7.14 Hamartoma. These lesions consist of an admixture of tissue elements normally found in the breast (i.e., fat, fibrous tissue, glandular structures, and, in some cases, smooth muscle). In this particular case, the smooth muscle component is particularly prominent (inset), and such lesions are designated "myoid hamartomas."

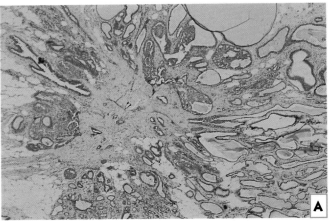

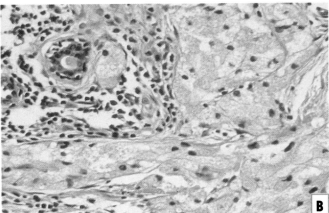

Figure 7.15 Radial scar. (A) Low-power view demonstrates a stellate lesion with a central fibroelastotic core surrounded by ducts which appear to radiate from it. (B) Higher-power view shows that the central core contains entrapped, benign epithelial elements. Some of the surrounding ducts show intraductal hyperplasia.

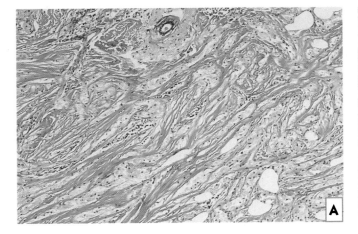

Figure 7.16 Granular cell tumor. (A) Low-power view showing tumor cells embedded in a dense fibrotic stroma. (B) At higher power the tumor cells show small, uniform nuclei and abundant, finely granular eosinophilic cytoplasm. These lesions are ty benign.

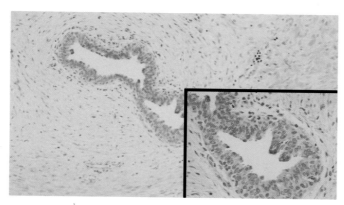

Figure 7.17 Gynecomastia. The breast tissue is composed of ducts that show varying degrees of epithelial hyperplasia. The ducts are surrounded by loose, moderately cellular connective tissue (inset). Lobular development is usually not observed.

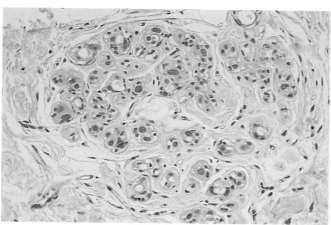

Figure 7.18 Radiation effect. This terminal duct lobular unit shows atrophic changes and scattered atypical epithelial cells with large nuclei. This combination of features is characteristic of radiation effect and can be seen to some degree in virtually all patients who have received therapeutic doses of ionizing radiation. In some cases these terminal duct lobular unit changes are accompanied by epithelial atypia in larger (extralobular) ducts, stromal changes (hyalinization, atypical fibroblasts), and vascular changes such as myointimal hyperplasia of small arteries and endothelial cell atypia. Similar changes in the terminal ducts and lobules have been noted in patients treated with chemotherapy.

SUGGESTED READING

Consensus Meeting. (1986) Is "fibrocystic disease" of the breast precancerous? *Arch Pathol Lab Med* 110:171–173.

Dupont WD, Page DL. (1985) Risk factors for breast cancer in women with proliferative breast disease. *N Engl J Med* 312:146–151.

Hayes DF. (1991) Breast cancer. In: Skarin AT, ed. *Atlas of Diagnostic Oncology*. New York: Gower Medical Publishing, 6.1–6.31.

Page DL, Dupont WD, Rogers LW, Rados MS. (1985) Atypical hyperplastic lesions of the female breast: a long-term follow-up study. *Cancer* 55:2698–2708.

Page DL. (1986) Cancer risk assessment in benign breast biopsies. *Hum Pathol* 17:871–874.

Schnitt SJ, Connolly JL. (1991) Pathology of benign breast disorders. In: Harris JR, Hellman S, Henderson IC, Kinne DW, eds. *Breast Diseases*, 2nd ed. Philadelphia: JB Lippincott, 15–30.

Schnitt SJ, Connolly JL, Harris J, Cohen R. (1984) Radiation-induced changes in the breast. *Hum Pathol* 15:545–550.

The invasive breast carcinomas also comprise a heterogeneous group of lesions. The most common type is infiltrating ductal carcinoma (also termed infiltrating carcinoma of no special type or infiltrating carcinoma, not otherwise specified). These tumors are usually hard, gray, gritty masses that invade the surrounding tissue (Fig. 8.5). On microscopic examination, infiltrating ductal carcinomas are divided into three grades—well-differentiated (grade I), moderately differentiated (grade II), and poorly differentiated (grade III)—based on a combination of architectural and cytologic features (Fig. 8.6). The prognostic significance of this grading system has been repeatedly documented in clinical follow-up studies. Approximately 20 percent of invasive breast cancers are considered "special types." Infiltrating lobular carcinomas are the second most common type of invasive breast cancer (Fig. 8.7). These tumors have a higher frequency of bilaterality and multicentricity than infiltrating ductal carcinomas. Although some authors have reported that the prognosis for infiltrating lobular cancers is similar to that of invasive ductal lesions, others believe that the classical cases of infiltrating lobular carcinomas with low-grade nuclei are a prognostically favorable subset. Other variants of invasive breast carcinoma, such as medullary, mucinous (colloid), tubular, and papillary carcinomas, all have a better prognosis than infiltrat-

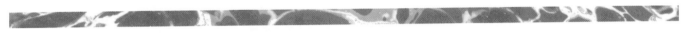

Figure 8.4 Histologic Subtypes of Ductal Carcinoma in Situ

	Comedo	Noncomedo
Cytology	High grade	Low grade
Proliferative rate	High	Low
Aneuploidy	Frequent	Infrequent
Her-2/*neu* oncogene expression	Frequent	Infrequent
Microinvasion	More common	Less common
Mammographic calcifications	Linear, branching ("casting")	Punctate

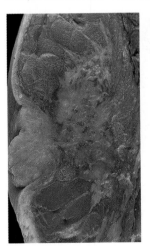

Figure 8.5 Macroscopic appearance of an infiltrating ductal carcinoma in a mastectomy specimen. The lesion is firm and shows extensions into the adjacent fat. This macroscopic appearance has been termed "scirrhous." (From Hayes, 1991.)

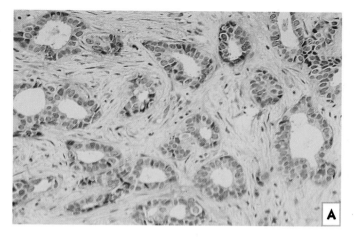

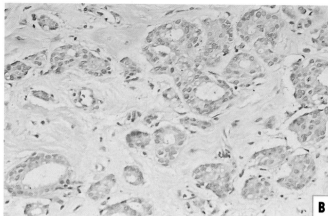

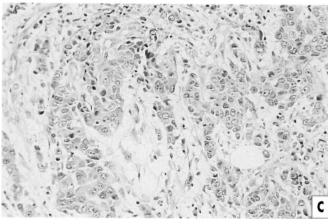

Figure 8.6 Infiltrating ductal carcinoma. (A) Well-differentiated (grade I). The tumor cells grow in glandular configurations. (B) Moderately differentiated (grade II). There is a mixture of well-formed glands and more solid tumor cell nests. (C) Poorly differentiated (grade III). The tumor is composed entirely of solid nests of tumor cells without evidence of gland formation.

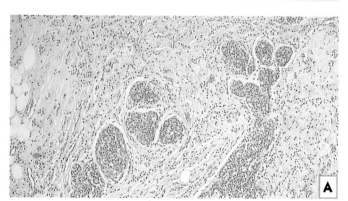

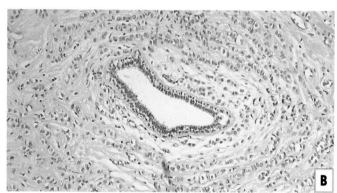

Figure 8.7 Infiltrating lobular carcinoma (classical type). (A) This tumor is characterized by small tumor cells that infiltrate the stroma in a single-file pattern. (B) The tumor cells in this section grow in a target-like pattern around a normal breast duct. (From Hayes, 1991.)

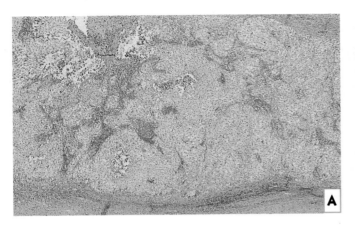

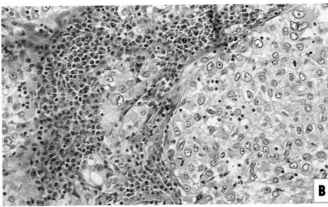

Figure 8.8 Medullary carcinoma. This type of breast carcinoma is characterized by macroscopic and microscopic circumscription, poorly differentiated (high-grade) tumor cells that grow in a syncytial pattern, and a diffuse lymphoplasmacytic infiltrate.

(A) Low-power photomicrograph demonstrates circumscribed tumor border. (B) High-power view demonstrates large, pleomorphic tumor cells and associated lymphocytes and plasma cells.

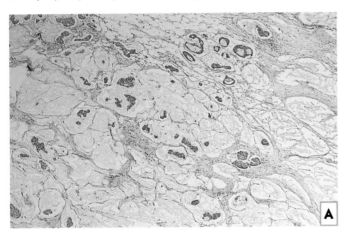

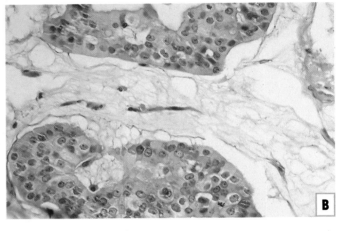

Figure 8.9 Mucinous (colloid) carcinoma. (A) Low-power view demonstrates islands of tumor cells within a sea of mucin. (B) Higher magnification shows tumor cell nests. The cells compris-

ing this type of tumor are typically rather uniform in appearance. (From Hayes, 1991.)

Figure 8.10 Tubular carcinoma. This type of breast cancer is composed of tubular structures infiltrating the stroma. The tubules tend to be elongated, and many have pointed ends. The cells composing the tubules are cuboidal to columnar and often have apical cytoplasmic protrusions or "snouts." (From Hayes, 1991.)

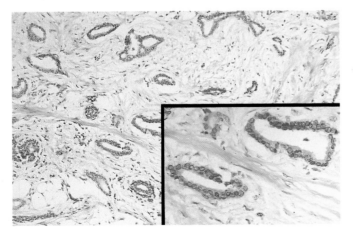

ing ductal carcinomas (Figs. 8.8–8.10). More unusual variants of invasive breast cancer include metaplastic carcinomas (Fig. 8.11) and adenoid cystic carcinomas (Fig. 8.12). The frequency of the more common types of invasive breast carcinoma in two large studies is shown in Figure 8.13.

A number of histologic features of breast carcinomas have been reported to be associated with an unfavorable prognosis. These include lymphatic vessel and blood vessel invasion, tumor necrosis, and a prominent lymphoplasmacytic infiltrate (for nonmedullary types), among others (Fig. 8.14). An extensive intraductal component within an infiltrating ductal carcinoma has been associated with an increased risk of tumor recurrence in the breast after conservative surgery and radiation therapy (see Chapter 9).

A few types of breast carcinoma merit special attention. Paget's disease is a disorder of the nipple and areola, characterized clinically by an eczematoid appearance with crusting, scaling, or erosion. Histologically, breast cancer cells are found within the nipple and the areolar epidermis (Fig. 8.15). This lesion is almost always asso-

ciated with an underlying mammary carcinoma, which may be either in situ or invasive. Inflammatory carcinoma is a form of locally advanced breast cancer characterized clinically by erythema, edema, and warmth of the skin of the breast. Histopathologic examination of the skin typically demonstrates dermal lymphatic invasion by tumor cells (Fig. 8.16).

OTHER BREAST NEOPLASMS

Phyllodes tumors (cystosarcoma phyllodes) are tumors composed of a mixture of hypercellular stroma and benign ductal structures. The stroma is the neoplastic element in these tumors, and it may be cytologically bland or frankly sarcomatous (Fig. 8.17). Angiosarcomas are uncommon malignant vascular tumors. These lesions, particularly when of high grade, are extremely aggressive (Fig. 8.18). Other types of sarcomas may arise in the breast but are extremely rare. Lymphomas may involve the breast either as primary tumors or in conjunction with lymphoma in extramammary sites (Fig. 8.19).

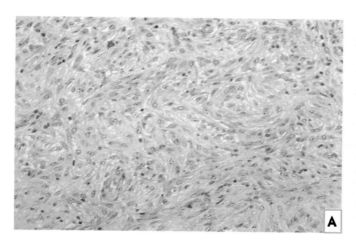

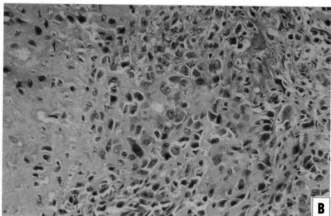

Figure 8.11 Metaplastic carcinomas. These are unusual variants of invasive breast cancers in which the tumor cells are of a type other than the glandular cells that comprise the common types of breast cancer. Tumor cells may be squamous, spindle-shaped, or may form cartilage or bone. (A) Metaplastic carcinoma composed primarily of spindle cells. (B) Metaplastic carcinoma with differentiation toward cartilage. Tumors with spindle cell morphology have a prognosis similar to that of infiltrating ductal carcinoma. Metaplastic carcinomas with heterologous elements (e.g., malignant cartilage or bone) have a poorer prognosis.

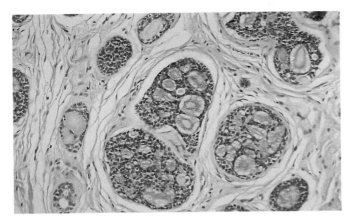

Figure 8.12 Adenoid cystic carcinoma. This type of invasive cancer is characterized by tumor cell nests containing glandular spaces. Within many of the gland lumina are hyaline deposits. These tumors have a better prognosis than the usual infiltrating ductal carcinomas.

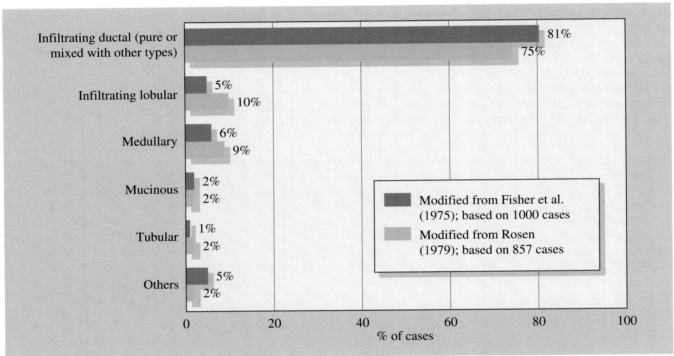

Figure 8.13 Frequency of histologic types of invasive breast cancer in two large series.

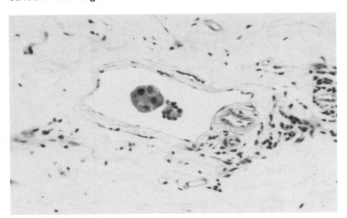

Figure 8.14 Lymphatic vessel invasion adversely affects the prognosis in patients with invasive breast cancer.

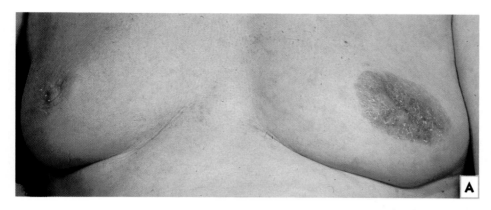

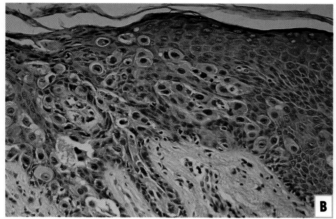

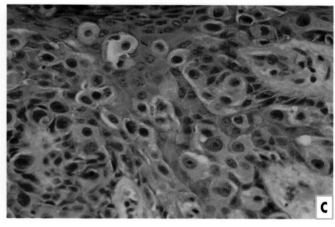

Figure 8.15 Paget's disease. Clinically, patients with this disorder present with an eczematous lesion of the nipple that may also involve the areola. This lesion is typically associated with an underlying breast cancer. (A) Photograph demonstrates eczema-toid change of the left nipple and areola. (From Hayes, 1991.) (B) The epidermis is infiltrated by cancer cells with abundant pink cytoplasm and large, vesicular nuclei with prominent nucleoli. (C) High-power view demonstrates tumor cells within the epidermis.

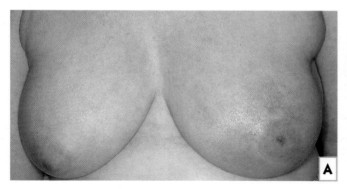

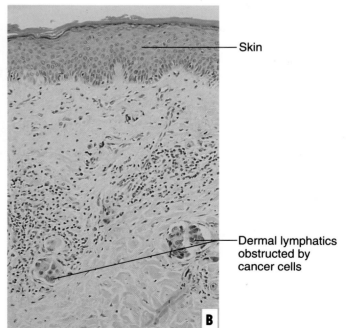

Skin

Dermal lymphatics obstructed by cancer cells

Figure 8.16 Inflammatory carcinoma. (A) Classically, inflammatory breast cancer does not present as a discrete mass, but rather as cutaneous erythema with overlying skin warmth, as illustrated in the left breast of this 63-year-old patient. (B) Pathologic confirmation of invasion of dermal lymphatics by malignant cells, as shown in this photomicrograph, can help distinguish this condition from benign mastitis. The erythema and warmth observed clinically are due to obstruction of dermal lymphatics and subsequent cutaneous lymphedema. (From Hayes, 1991.)

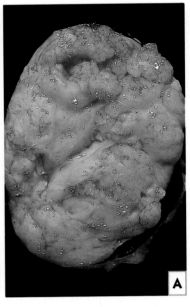

Figure 8.17 Phyllodes tumor (cystosarcoma phyllodes). (A) These lesions are circumscribed masses which, on cut surface, show cleft-like spaces intermingled with tan–yellow nodules of tumor. (From Hayes, 1991.) (B) Low-power microscopic examination reveals that the tumor is composed primarily of hypercellular stroma. A benign ductal structure is also seen. (C) High-power view shows atypical stromal cells with one mitotic figure. The stroma may be benign or malignant. When malignant, the stroma may be composed of fibrosarcoma, liposarcoma, chondrosarcoma, osteosarcoma, or rhabdomyosarcoma.

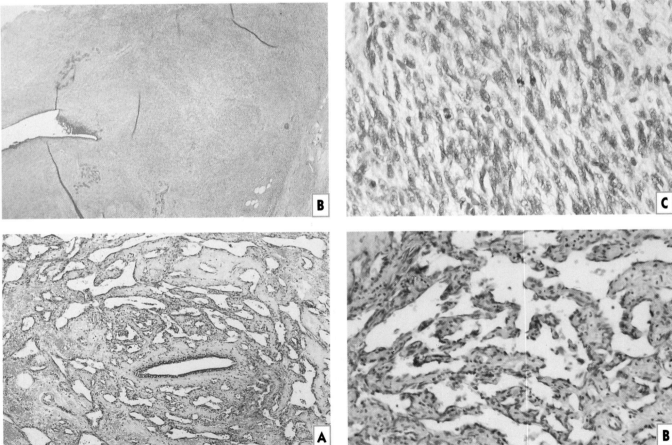

Figure 8.18 Angiosarcoma. (A) In this relatively well-differentiated angiosarcoma, interanastomosing vascular spaces infiltrate the breast stroma. (B) Higher-power view shows papillary projections of malignant endothelial cells within the vascular spaces.

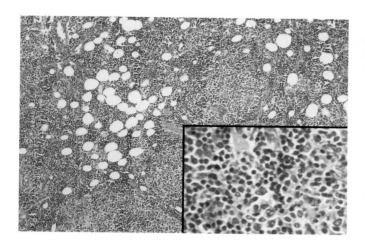

Figure 8.19 Lymphoma. The breast tissue is infiltrated by atypical lymphoid cells in a nodular and diffuse pattern. The inset shows an example of a follicular center cell lymphoma, mixed small-cell and large cell type.

SUGGESTED READING

Fisher ER, Gregorio RM, Fisher B, et al. (1975) The pathology of invasive breast cancer. A syllabus derived from findings from the National Surgical Adjuvant Breast Project (Protocol #4). *Cancer* 36:1–85.

Hayes DF. (1991) Breast cancer. In Skarin AT, ed. *Atlas of Diagnostic Oncology*. New York: Gower Medical Publishing, 6.1–6.31.

Page DL. (1991) Prognosis and breast cancer. Recognition of lethal and favorable prognostic types. *Am J Surg Pathol* 15:334–349.

Rosen PP. (1979) The pathological classification of human mammary carcinoma: Past, present and future. *Ann Clin Lab Sci* 9:144–156.

Rosen PP. (1991) The pathology of invasive breast carcinoma. In Harris JR, Hellman S, Henderson IC, Kinne DW, eds. *Breast Diseases* (2nd ed). Philadelphia: JB Lippincott, 245–296.

Schnitt SJ. (1991) Pathology of in situ carcinoma. In Harris JR, Hellman S, Henderson IC, Kinne DW, eds. *Breast Diseases* (2nd ed). Philadelphia: JB Lippincott, 229–232.

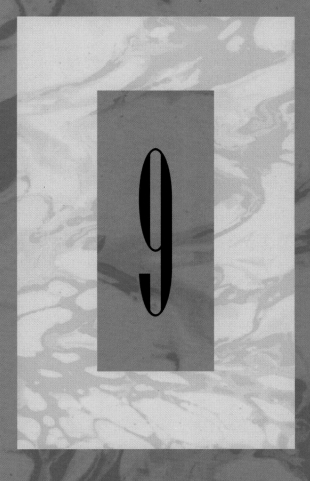

9

Radiotherapy Techniques

Abram Recht

The breast-conserving treatment of early-stage breast carcinoma at present employs a combination of conservative surgery (CS) for resection of the primary tumor with a surrounding margin of grossly normal breast tissue ("lumpectomy," "partial mastectomy," "segmental mastectomy," or "quadrantectomy"), with or without surgical staging of the axillary nodes and radiation therapy (RT) for the eradication of residual subclinical disease. The goal of such treatment is to provide highly satisfactory cosmetic results without compromise of local tumor control or survival. Cooperation among the surgeon, radiologist, pathologist, medical oncologist, and radiation oncologist is critical in obtaining good results with CS and RT.

Large, randomized controlled trials have demonstrated that treatment of carefully selected patients with CS and RT yields a survival rate equal to that of mastectomy, with the advantage of organ preservation (Fig. 9.1). A conference convened by the National Cancer Institute (U.S.) concluded that "breast conservation treatment is an appropriate method of primary therapy for the majority of women with Stage I and II breast cancer, and preferable because it provides survival equiv-

alent to total mastectomy and also preserves the breast."

The success of breast-conserving therapy depends on two factors: appropriate selection of patients who are and are not candidates for treatment by CS and RT, and proper implementation of the available treatment techniques.

SELECTION OF PATIENTS FOR TREATMENT WITH CS AND RT

The major criteria for patient selection for CS and RT are: the ability to resect the primary malignancy without causing major cosmetic deformities and the likelihood of tumor recurrence (especially in comparison with the local–regional failure rate of mastectomy). Although the impact on survival of locally recurrent breast carcinoma after conservative therapy is unclear, such recurrence defeats a major goal of conservative treatment, namely the preservation of the breast. In addition, recurrence of breast cancer is an enormously traumatic event from the psychologic standpoint. Therefore, the possibility of local recurrence must be minimized by careful attention to patient selection and treatment.

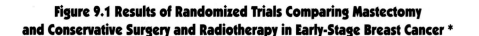

Figure 9.1 Results of Randomized Trials Comparing Mastectomy and Conservative Surgery and Radiotherapy in Early-Stage Breast Cancer *

Trial	# Pts	FU (mo)	Survival at	Mast. Arm	CS & RT Arm
Milan	701	Min 120	10 yr	76%	79%
WHO	179	Mean 120	10 yr	80%	79%
NSABP	1219	Mean 81	8 yr	71%	76%
NCI, U.S.	237	Med 68	8 yr	79%	85%
Denmark	859	Med 40	6 yr	82%	79%
EORTC	874	Min 36	?	←———— Equal ————→	

*From Fisher and Redmond (1992); van Dongen, Bartelink, Fentiman, et al. (1992); Blichert-Toft, Rose, Andersen, et al. (1992); and Straus, Lichter, Lippman, et al. (1992).

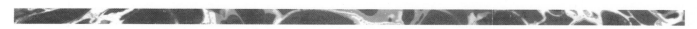

Three factors must considered when patients are evaluated as potential candidates for breast-conserving therapy: patient factors, clinical factors, and pathologic factors (Fig. 9.2).

Patient Factors

The only absolute contraindication to RT treatment of patients with operable breast cancer is pregnancy, as substantial risks to the fetus (tumor induction, microcephaly, and other congenital anomalies) cannot be avoided. Patient preference for mastectomy or breast-conserving treatment will otherwise dictate management, assuming that the physician believes the cure rate likely to be equal with either approach. Other patient factors are of less importance in guiding treatment selection.

Past experience initially suggested that patients younger than 35 to 40 years of age at diagnosis had a higher risk than older patients of breast tumor recurrence after CS and RT. However, this marked disparity in results has recently been substantially reduced or eliminated by improvements in evaluation and surgical techniques. Although elderly patients may have more severe logistical problems in coping with a six-week course of daily RT than younger individuals, acute or chronic reactions to treatment are not significantly worse than those of younger patients. Certain coexisting medical problems, especially collagen vascular diseases, may adversely affect the cosmetic results of RT and increase the risk of complications. Other medical problems do not noticeably affect the outcome of treatment with CS and RT, but in practice may make the use of RT impractical (e.g., nonambulatory patients).

Clinical Factors

The ability to perform a cosmetically satisfactory resection of a primary breast tumor depends on the size and location of the tumor, the size of the breast, and the extent of the surgical margin felt to be necessary.

Unless the patient has large breasts, it is usually difficult to perform an acceptable resection for a tumor greater than 4–5 cm in diameter. Women with small, average, and large breasts may be treated with excellent cosmetic results, although large-breasted women may be at greater risk for developing breast retraction.

The presence of nipple discharge, especially in association with a central lesion, may indicate involvement of the nipple–areola complex. Resection of the nipple and areola may be necessay for adequate treatment of these women, and the cosmetic results may not be acceptable to the patient.

Patients with multiple lesions on palpation or radiologic evidence of diffuse or multicentric disease are usually not good candidates for CS and RT, as they have a substantial risk of local failure.

Histopathologic Factors

Patients in whom gross residual disease remains after initial biopsy have a substantially greater risk of local failure than patients in whom a gross total excision is performed; therefore, re-excision is necessary in such patients. However, the importance of microscopic mar-

Figure 9.2 Factors To Consider in Evaluating Patients for Treatment with Breast-conserving Therapy*

Patient Factors	Clinical Factors	Histopathologic Factors
Pregnancy	Tumor size in relation to breast size	Presence and extent of microscopic involvement of resection margins
Patient preference	Presence of nipple discharge	Histologic features of the tumor
Age	Tumor location	
Collagen vascular diseases	Presence of multiple lesions on palpation	
Other medical conditions	Radiologic evidence of diffuse or multi centric disease	

*Modified from Recht and Harris (1990).

gin involvement by tumor has not been established. One reason for this uncertainty is that there are technical problems in assessing the margins. Proper handling of surgical specimens is discussed in Chapter 6. Recent data suggest that the use of a "boost" dose of radiation to the tumor bed, in addition to irradition of the entire breast, yields a high level of local control even when microscopic resection margins are positive.

In patients whose infiltrating ductal carcinomas are treated by a simple gross excision of the tumor, one important factor that predicts an increased likelihood of tumor recurrence is the presence of an extensive intraductal carcinoma component (EIC). An EIC-positive tumor is defined by the presence of two features: intraductal carcinoma comprising a prominent portion of the area of the primary mass, and intraductal carcinoma clearly extending beyond the infiltrating margin of the

tumor or present in sections of grossly normal adjacent breast tissue. Predominantly noninvasive tumors, with only focal areas of invasion, are also included in this category. In patients who are EIC-positive, the actuarial risk of breast recurrence is 24 percent at 5 years and 32 percent at 10 years, compared with only 6 percent at 5 years and 14 percent at 10 years for other patients (Fig. 9.3).

The reason for the association of EIC with a high risk of local recurrence is not entirely clear. It seems probable that these patients have a greater residual tumor burden after gross excision than do other patients. Therefore, the optimal extent of resection may depend on the extent of associated intraductal carcinoma. Evaluation of patients after initial excision can proceed as suggested. Patients without EIC are well treated by excisional biopsy with narrow gross tissue margins. When the margins are heavily involved or cannot be

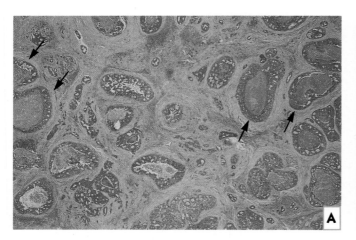

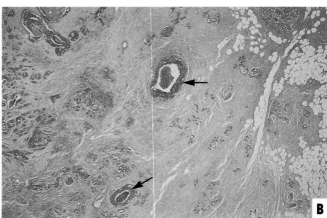

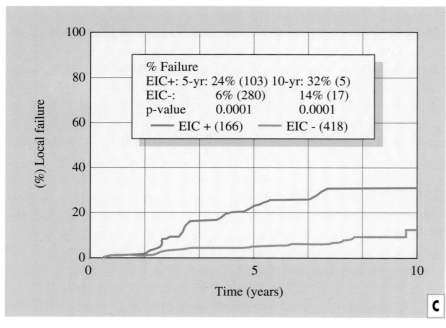

Figure 9.3 (A,B) Extensive introductal component. This tumor is principally an invasive ductal carcinoma. However, a prominent intraductal component (arrows) is present within the invasive tissue (A), as well as in the surrounding normal parenchyma (B). (Arrows demonstrate intraductal component.) (C) Breast recurrence in patients with or without an extensive intraductal carcinoma component (EIC). Results from the JCRT in patients treated from 1982–1985 showed that the presence or absence of an EIC was the single most important factor in predicting the risk of local recurrence in patients with infiltrating ductal carcinomas treated with simple gross excision of the tumor and RT. (From Boyages, Recht, Connolly, et al. (1990); with permission.)

evaluated, a re-excision should be performed before implementation of RT. In patients with EIC, the specimen and mammograms should be carefully reviewed to be certain that the areas of intraductal spread have been adequately excised. Postoperative mammograms may be helpful in this regard (see Chapter 4). When EIC is present and the margins are microscopically involved or equivocal, the biopsy site should be re-excised. (See Chapter 6 for a discussion of margin assessment.) A cosmetically and pathologically satisfactory re-excision can be achieved in most patients. If the margins of the re-excision specimen are also involved, then the patient should be told that she may still be at greater risk of local recurrence if treated by radiotherapy than if treated by mastectomy, despite the re-excision. Although the rates of distant metastases and survival to date have been the same in groups both at low and at high risk of breast recurrence, this may change with further follow-up, and hence mastectomy may be preferable. In addition, when re-excision is not technically possible or cannot be done without severe deformity of the breast, mastectomy may be more desirable.

It has also become apparent that modern film-screen mammography is an extremely valuable tool both in pretreatment evaluation of patients considered for CS and RT and in their follow-up handling (see Chapter 4). Magnification views are especially helpful in delineating unsuspected tumor extension, and postoperative mammography can be very useful for assessment of the completeness of surgical resection.

COSMETIC RESULTS OF TREATMENT

The cosmetic results after treatment with CS and RT are usually good to excellent, and almost all patients are satisfied with the results (Fig. 9.4). Overall cosmetic results decline during the first three years after treatment but then remain stable. Several factors are associated with a poor outcome (Fig. 9.5): greater breast size; large tumor size; extensive surgical resection; a three-field radiotherapy technique; the use of large RT fraction sizes; the use of an iridium-192 implant; and the use of chemotherapy, especially when given concurrently with irradiation.

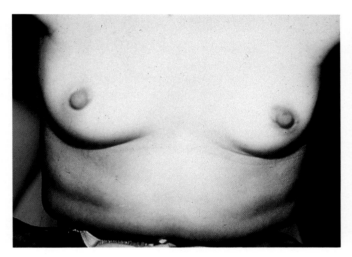

Figure 9.4 Excellent cosmetic results in a patient with small breasts. Can you determine which side was treated?

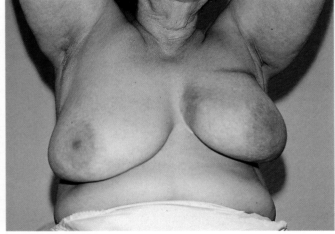

Figure 9.5 Poor cosmetic result in a patient with large breasts resulting from substantial retraction and fibrosis. Patients with large breasts tend to have more retraction after CS and RT than those with moderate or small breasts, but this risk can be reduced by careful attention to treatment technique. This patient was treated with the "hockey-stick" technique. Note lines of hyperpigmentation superiorly and medially to the left breast. These are areas in which the hockey-stick and tangential field overlapped. On palpation, these areas have increased induration compared to the breast.

TREATMENT OF THE REGIONAL LYMPH NODES

The utility of treating the regional lymph nodes as part of the overall management of patients undergoing CS and RT is controversial. However, either axillary dissection or axillary irradiation can achieve regional tumor control in almost all patients who present without clinically suspicious axillary adenopathy. Therefore, it is controversial whether all patients treated with CS and RT require an axillary dissection. However, axillary dissection yields information concerning the prognosis and the risk of involvement of the internal mammary and supraclavicular regions. At present, the results of axillary dissection are also used to help determine the role and type of adjuvant systemic therapy. Radiotherapy treatment to the breast alone after axillary dissection is acceptable in all situations. Nevertheless, it is reasonable to treat the axillary, supraclavicular, and/or internal mammary node areas in selected high-risk patients. Figure 9.6 contains possible guidelines to the management of the regional nodes.

COMPLICATIONS OF TREATMENT

Complications resulting from RT can be divided into acute reactions (during and shortly after treatment) and chronic complications (not usually appearing until months or years after treatment (Figs. 9.7–9.12). The incidence of such complications depends greatly on the treatment techniques used (both surgical and radiotherapeutic) and on whether adjuvant chemo-therapy is given as well. For example, the incidence of radiation pneumonitis depends both upon the sequencing of

Figure 9.6 Guidelines on Treatment of Regional Lymph Nodes*

Nonpalpable (N0) Axillary Nodes	Palpable (N1) Axillary Nodes	Axillary or Supraclavicular Radiotherapy
Axillary dissection preferred	Axillary dissection should be performed	Should not routinely be given following adequate axillary dissection (i.e., removal of level I/II nodes) when the nodes are negative or only 1–3 nodes are positive.
If dissection not performed, treat axillary nodes with RT		Insufficient data at present to justify firm recommendations regarding axillary and supraclavicular irradiation for patients with four or more positive nodes. The benefits of such treatment, if any, are likely to be small.
		Whether some subgroups (e.g., patients with greater than 50% of the removed nodes involved or extensive extracapsular spread of disease) might benefit more than others from treatment of the regional nodes is unknown.

*Modified from Recht, Pierce, Abner, et al. (1991).

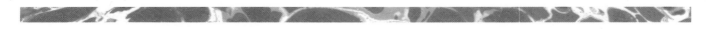

Figure 9.7 Possible Complications After CS and RT When Nodal RT Is Included

Immediate Reactions

Common

Skin reddening and irritation

Skin darkening

Tiredness

Decreased blood cell count

Occasional aches and pains in the breast

Temporary hair loss in the treated area

Uncommon

Skin blistering

Nausea

Long-term Reactions

Common

Occasional discomfort and sensitivity in the treated area

Mild to moderately increased firmness of the treated breast

Mild swelling of the treated breast, which can last for a number of years

Minor shrinkage of the treated breast

Uncommon

Rib fractures in the treated area

Significant increase in firmness of the treated breast

Increased risk of swelling of arm

Significant shrinkage of the treated breast

Rare

Lung inflammation and scarring

Damage to nerves to the arm

Extremely rare

Inflammation of the lining of the heart or heart attack (only if left breast treated)

New tumor in the treated area or other breast or leukemia

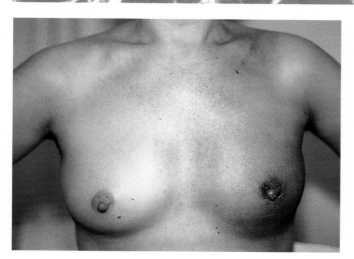

Figure 9.8 Acute skin reaction (erythema), after completing radiotherapy. The acute skin erythema and dry desquammation will heal within two to three weeks. Note the hyperpigmentation of the skin and nipple-areola complex. This will gradually fade over six to 12 months.

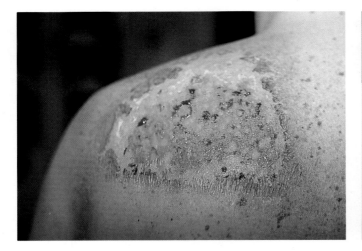

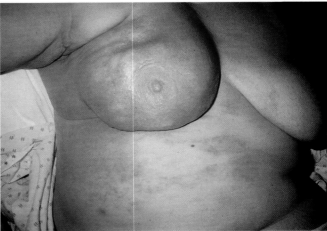

Figure 9.9 "Recall reaction." Moist desquammation developing in area of exit from supraclavicular/axillary field due to administration of doxorubicin-containing chemotherapy following radiotherapy. The exact mechanism by which anthracyclines can cause such a delayed skin reaction is unknown. Both acute and chronic complications may be increased in frequency and severity when chemotherapy is used as well as CS and RT.

Figure 9.10 Episode of acute cellulitis developing in the breast six years after treatment with CS and RT. Note the spread of the infection to the unirradiated chest and also to the abdominal wall inferiorly. Such occurrences are fortunately very rare, and usually occur in patients who have had substantial fibrosis and compromise of the skin, as is seen in this patient.

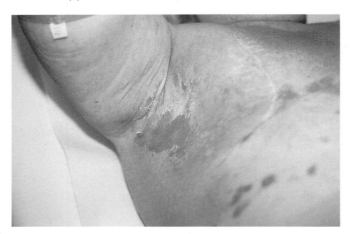

Figure 9.11 Moist desquammation in a patient undergoing postmastectomy RT at 38 Gy. Because of the need to treat the skin and subcutaneous tissues, patients treated with RT after mastectomy usually have a more pronounced acute skin reaction than patients treated with CS and RT. A short "break" from treatment may be needed to allow healing to begin. However, such reactions rarely lead to infection, and they heal completely within a few weeks after completion of RT.

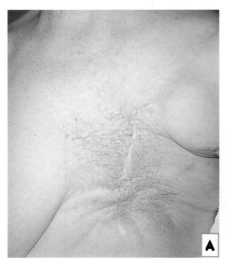
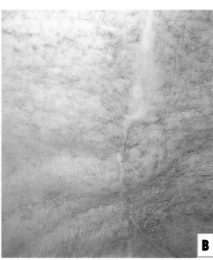

Figure 9.12 Severe telangectasias following postmastectomy chest-wall RT. (A) Entire chest wall. (B) Close-up view. Telangectasias may take four to five years to reach maximum intensity. In addition, patients may have some degree of cutaneous fibrosis. However, these changes rarely lead to functional limitations or other problems.

chemotherapy and RT and on the volume of lung tissue treated. Similarly, the incidence of brachial plexopathy not only depends on the total dose of RT given but may also depend on whether chemotherapy is given.

The most feared complication of radiotherapy is the induction of second tumors, particularly sarcomas (Fig. 9.13). Fortunately these seem very rare. The incidence of sarcomas was 2/2850 (21.9 per 100,00 patient-years observation) in patients surviving at least five years after treatment with CS and RT at the Marseille Cancer Institute.

RADIOTHERAPY TECHNIQUES

The radiation oncologist should optimize techniques and doses of RT in order to minimize the risk of local recurrence, achieve excellent cosmetic results, and avoid both short- and long-term complications (Figs. 9.14–9.19). It is uncertain whether the entire breast should be treated or only a more limited volume surrounding the tumor. Most radiation oncologists treat the entire breast. Doses higher than 50 Gy (delivered in daily treatments over five weeks) cause significant breast retraction and fibrosis.

Similarly, the need for a radiation boost dose to the primary site is also controversial (Fig. 9.20). As noted, the utility of a boost must be considered in relation to the extent of surgical resection. It is probable that a boost is more important after routine excisional biopsy than after very wide excision or quadrantectomy. Nevertheless, the morbidity of a boost of moderate size and dose is small. Therefore, the combination of local excision and radiotherapy including a boost provides both an excellent level of local tumor control and

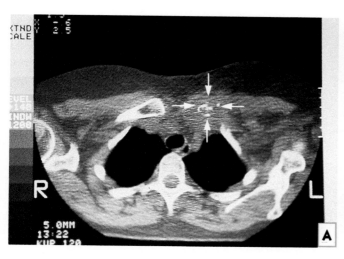

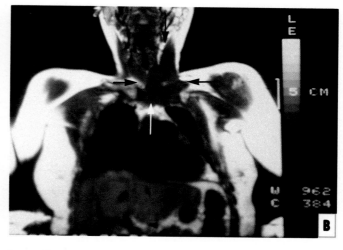

Figure 9.13 Malignant fibrous histiocytoma of the clavicle nine years after CS and RT. (A) Transverse CT scan. (B) Coronal MRI image. Tumor is identified by arrows. Note extensive infiltration into the adjacent soft tissues. The most feared complication of RT is a radiation-induced tumor. These may occur as early as four years after RT or ≥30 years later. The prognosis of patients with such lesions is dismal. Fortunately, such tumors are rare.

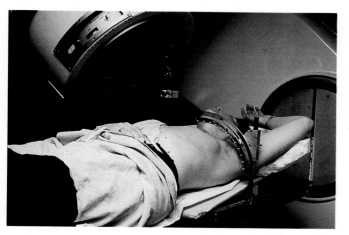

Figure 9.14 Patient being set up for external-beam RT on treatment accelerator. She lies supine with her arm above her head and is positioned reproducibly each day with the aid of laser pointers and skin tattoos. A "protractor" (curved metal device on the edge of the treatment couch) is used to accurately match the breast tangential fields and the supraclavicular or supraclavicular–axillary field (see Fig. 9.15).

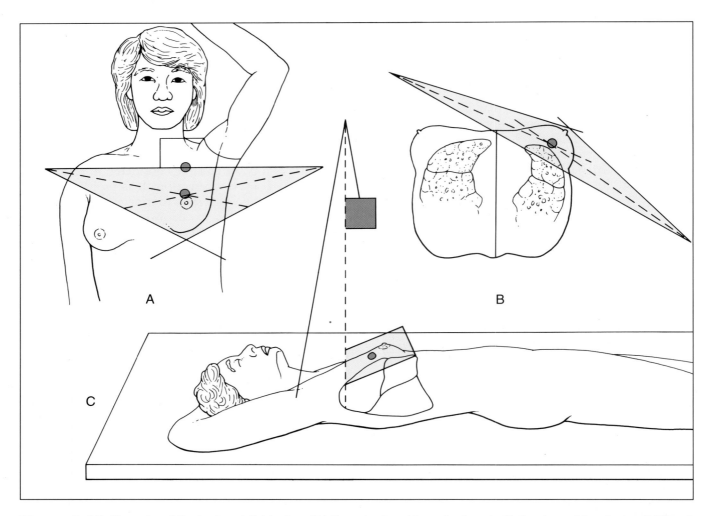

Figure 9.15 Geometry of the treatment field setup. (A) The breast is treated with tangential fields that enter at the midaxillary line and exit at the midline or several cm across the midline. (B) The gantry is angled to align the posterior field edges, to minimize the amount of lung treated. (C) The collimator that defines the treatment beam is aligned with the slope of the chest wall. When it is desirable to treat the supraclavicular and axillary nodes, it is necessary to use a "third" field directed toward these areas (see A). To avoid overlap between these fields, a "corner-block technique" is used to match field edges together (see C).

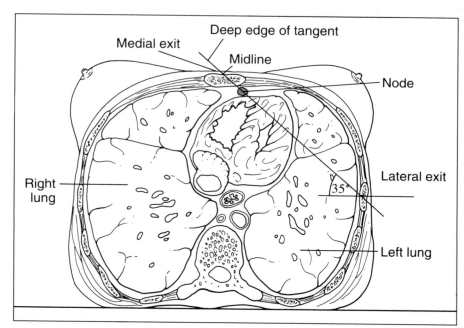

Deep edge of tangent

Medial exit

Midline

Node

Right lung

Lateral exit

35°

Left lung

Figure 9.16 Transverse section showing organs irradiated when tangential fields are treated, with medial and lateral exit points of fields noted. Observe the location of the internal mammary node in proximity to the heart.

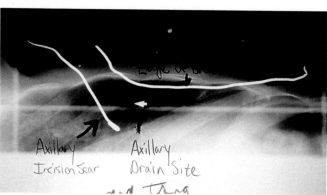

Axillary Incision Scar   Axillary Drain Site

Figure 9.17 Radiograph ("simulator film") taken at the time of treatment planning for tangential breast treatment. The relationship of the treatment fields to the lateral edge of the breast tissue, the axillary dissection scar, and an axillary drain site is demonstrated.

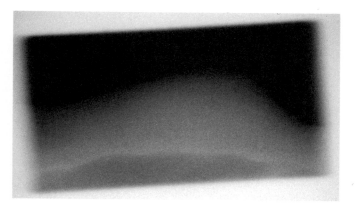

Figure 9.18 Radiograph taken on the linear accelerator, or "port film." This is compared to the simulator film to confirm that the patient is correctly positioned, that the treatment fields are of the correct size, and that blocks are correctly placed.

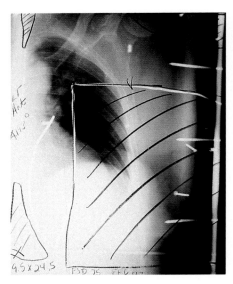

Figure 9.19 "Hockey-stick" technique. One external-beam treatment approach used in the past has been to use a single photon field to treat the axillary, supraclavicular, and internal mammary nodes, and tangential fields to treat the breast. This simulator film shows that a large volume of the lung and, for left-sided treatment, a large portion of the heart are included in the treatment area. This may lead to an increased risk of radiation-related pulmonary or cardiac complications. These complications can be largely avoided by the use of either electrons or a mixed electron-photon beam to treat the internal mammary nodes, or by including the internal mammary nodes in the tangential fields. Because one cannot simultaneously align all the edges of the tangential fields and the hockey-stick fields, there may also be significant overlap between field edges, producing poor cosmetic results or complications.

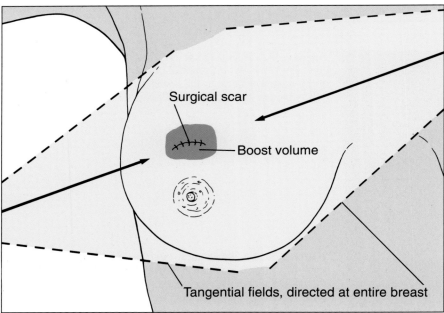

Surgical scar

Boost volume

Tangential fields, directed at entire breast

Figure 9.20 Schematic view of radiotherapy treatment strategy. The entire breast is treated to a moderate dose, using opposed fields tangential to the chest wall. An extra dose of radiation, or "boost," is then given to the tumor bed and its immediate vicinity, as the likelihood of having residual tumor (and its volume) is greater in this area than in other portions of the breast. The boost can be given with either external-beam radiotherapy (x-rays or electrons) or interstitial implantation. By giving different radiation doses to areas with different tumor burdens after surgery, this strategy maximizes local control while achieving excellent cosmetic results and low complication rates.

highly satisfactory cosmetic results. Randomized studies of this issue are presently being conducted. The boost dose is usually 10–20 Gy, or enough to bring the region of the tumor bed to a total dose of 60–65 Gy. Interstitial implantation and external-beam boosts (with photons or electrons) appear to yield equal local control and cosmetic results (Figs. 9.21 and 9.22).

Certain patients might be treated safely with CS alone with reasonably low breast recurrence rates. However, series of relatively unselected patients treated with CS without RT have reported local failure rates of 30 to 40 percent. Better results may be possible with careful preoperative evaluation, appropriate patient selection based on tumor size and histologic features, wide local excision, and painstaking histologic evaluation of resection margins. Survival is not clearly affected in patients who experience a higher incidence of breast recurrence, but studies of this issue are still in progress. CS alone should be used only as part of a well-defined protocol.

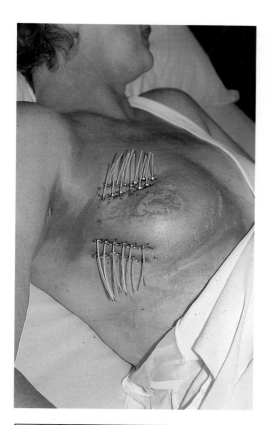

Figure 9.21 Iridium-192 interstitial implantation. This is used to give a boost dose of radiation to the site of the primary tumor after excision. In the operating room, stainless steel needles are inserted into the breast under either local or general anesthesia. Hollow plastic tubes are then slid into the needles, and the needles removed. Metal "buttons" are placed over the ends of the strands. After the patient returns to her room, thin radioactive wires are placed into the tube and the buttons are crimped, holding the implant securely in place. The implant is left in place from one to three days and is then removed at the bedside. Bleeding, infection, and other complications are rare. However, since equally good results can be obtained with external-beam boosts, the use of implants is now usually reserved for patients with unresectable lesions. (From Hayes, 1991.)

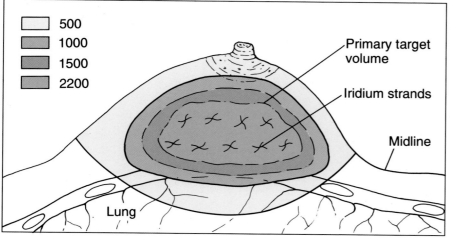

Figure 9.22 Example of a dose distribution around an iridium-192 interstitial breast implant.

RT AFTER MASTECTOMY

The role of RT after mastectomy is unclear. Although the use of postoperative RT clearly decreases the risk of local–regional recurrence, it is uncertain whether this will ultimately improve the survival rate. Multiple randomized prospective studies comparing patients treated with mastectomy only or with mastectomy and RT have not shown any significant survival advantage. However, these studies did not employ adjuvant systemic therapy. More recent studies have often shown an advantage in disease-free survival for patients who receive both RT and systemic treatment after mastectomy. These trials have insufficient follow-up as yet to determine whether overall survival will also be ultimately improved. Therefore, at present it seems reasonable to use RT after mastectomy in patients who have a very high risk of local–regional failure, such as those with locally advanced disease.

LOCALLY ADVANCED BREAST CANCER

Patients with locally advanced or unresectable breast cancer historically have been treated with RT alone, without either local excision or mastectomy. Very high RT doses can be given by using a combination of external beam and interstitial implantation. The cosmetic results of such treatment are usually acceptable, although not as good as those after CS and RT for earlier tumors (Fig. 9.23). However, local–regional failure

rates after radical RT alone have been from 25 to 50 percent, and may be even higher in patients with inflammatory breast cancer. As systemic therapy has improved, patients with locally advanced breast cancer are more commonly treated with a combined approach. In these cases, "up-front" or "neoadjuvant" chemotherapy and/or hormone therapy may reduce tumor bulk, perhaps allowing more effective local therapy with mastectomy and radiotherapy. Early results of this combined approach are promising.

LOCAL AND REGIONAL RECURRENCE AFTER MASTECTOMY OR CS AND RT

Recurrence After Mastectomy

The incidence of local–regional failure after mastectomy with histologically negative axillary nodes is from 3 to 8 percent. When the axillary lymph nodes are positive, however, the incidence increases to 19 to 27 percent. Most recurrences after mastectomy are on the chest wall (Fig. 9.24). Patients with locally advanced breast cancers have even higher local-regional failure rates after treatment with mastectomy. One-half to two-thirds of local–regional recurrences are the first or only site of recurrence; the remainder are simultaneous with or follow the development of distant metastases. Recurrences on the chest wall may cause pain or ulceration but are usually only mildly symptomatic. However,

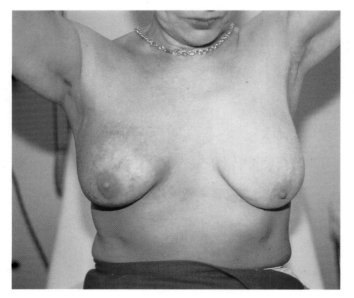

Figure 9.23 Cosmetic results five months after RT and chemotherapy without surgery for inflammatory breast cancer. The patient had a good cosmetic result but tumor recurred in the breast five years after treatment. She subsequently underwent mastectomy but developed distant metastases.

uncontrolled nodal recurrences commonly cause substantial arm edema, pain, and neurologic dysfunction (Figs. 9.25 and 9.26) (see also Chapter 5).

Despite aggressive local treatment, almost all patients with local–regional recurrence will eventually develop distant metastases. The median survival time for patients with isolated local recurrence is two to three years. However, only a fraction of these survivors will remain altogether free from further disease. RT can achieve permanent control of local–regional disease in only 40 to 60 percent of patients.

After Breast-conserving Therapy

The breast recurrence rate at five years for patients with early-stage cancers treated with CS and RT is 5 to 10 percent, with a 10-year recurrence rate of 7 to 20 percent. Recurrences have been seen as long as 21 years after CS and RT. The incidence of recurrence in the

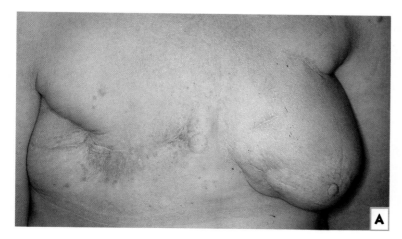

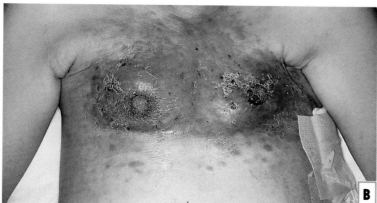

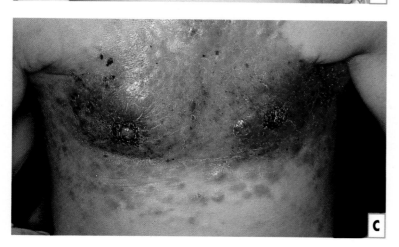

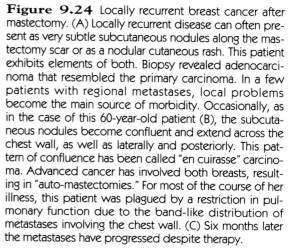

Figure 9.24 Locally recurrent breast cancer after mastectomy. (A) Locally recurrent disease can often present as very subtle subcutaneous nodules along the mastectomy scar or as a nodular cutaneous rash. This patient exhibits elements of both. Biopsy revealed adenocarcinoma that resembled the primary carcinoma. In a few patients with regional metastases, local problems become the main source of morbidity. Occasionally, as in the case of this 60-year-old patient (B), the subcutaneous nodules become confluent and extend across the chest wall, as well as laterally and posteriorly. This pattern of confluence has been called "en cuirasse" carcinoma. Advanced cancer has involved both breasts, resulting in "auto-mastectomies." For most of the course of her illness, this patient was plagued by a restriction in pulmonary function due to the band-like distribution of metastases involving the chest wall. (C) Six months later the metastases have progressed despite therapy.

breast in patients treated without excisional biopsy is substantially higher, as noted above. Approximately one-third of local recurrences are detected solely by follow-up mammography, one third on physical examination without any suspicious radiologic signs, and one-third are detected both by examination and mammography (see Chapter 4). The great majority of patients who present with a local relapse have recurrent tumor only in the breast parenchyma, without involvement of lymph nodes, skin, or the chest wall. Recurrence after CS and RT has a much better prognosis than local recurrence after mastectomy. It appears that a significant proportion of patients can be cured with salvage mastectomy, with long-term disease-free survival in about 50 percent of patients.

ROLE OF RT IN THE PALLIATION OF METASTATIC BREAST CANCER

RT has a substantial role in the palliation of metastatic breast cancer (see Chapter 13). The most common use of RT is for the treatment of bone metastases. Pain is completely or substantially relieved in 75 to 80 percent of patients who receive RT. Whether the use of RT reduces the likelihood of developing a pathologic fracture in a weight-bearing bone is not known. Many different fractionation schemes give equivalent results.

The most commonly employed regimens give 20 Gy in 5 fractions or 30 Gy in 10 fractions.

RT is also effective in reducing morbidity from metastases to other parts of the body. The results are often less rewarding than those achieved by treatment of bone metastases, however. The development of CNS metastases is a common problem, and RT provides very effective acute relief of symptoms in most patients. However, the median survival time for patients who develop brain metastases is less than six months. Unfortunately, many patients experience regrowth of their CNS lesions, because only rarely are they entirely eradicated. RT is also successful in the management of patients with spinal cord compression, with the results of treatment depending mainly on the patient's neurologic status at the time treatment is initiated.

CONCLUSIONS

Much has been learned about the management of patients with early-stage breast cancer. Still, controversial issues remain concerning patient selection and evaluation, and the optimal techniques of surgery and RT. In addition, further work is needed to clarify the best way to integrate CS and RT with adjuvant systemic treatment. The management of patients with ductal carcinoma in situ (DCIS) remains a major area of research.

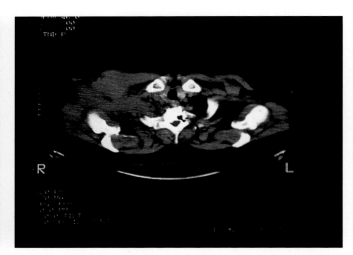

Figure 9.25 Axillary recurrence 18 months after left modified radical mastectomy. A 3-cm mass was palpable superior to the axillary extension of the mastectomy scar, under the edge of the pectoralis major muscle. The mass is indicated by the white circle. The lesion was resected and postoperative RT given.

Figure 9.26 Axillary recurrence after CS, axillary dissection, and breast RT. The patient presented with arm edema and paresthesias but no mass was palpable. CT showed extensive infiltration of the brachial plexus and encasement of the axillary vein. Bone metastases were also present. She had complete symptomatic relief and disappearence of arm edema after RT was given in conjunction with tamoxifen, but subsequently developed progressive bone disease.

SUGGESTED READING

Blichert-Toft N, Rose C, Andersen JA, et al. (1992) Danish randomized trial comparing breast conservation therapy with mastectomy: six years of life-table analysis. *J Natl Cancer Inst Monogr* 11:19–25.

Boyages J, Recht A, Connolly J, et al. (1990) Early breast cancer: Predictors of breast recurrence for patients treated with conservative surgery and radiation therapy. *Radiother Oncol* 19:29–41.

Fisher B, Redmond C. (1992) Lumpectomy for breast cancer: an update of the NSABP experience. *J Natl Cancer Inst Monogr* 11:7–13.

Harris JR, Hellman S, Henderson IC, Kinne DW. (1991) *Breast Diseases*. 2nd ed. Philadelphia: JB Lippincott, 1991.

Hayes DF. (1991) Breast cancer. In: Skarin AT, ed. *Atlas of Diagnostic Oncology*. New York: Gower Medical Publishing.

Kurtz JM, Amalric R, Delouche G, Pierquin B, Roth J, Spitalier J-M. (1987) The second ten years: Long-term risks of breast conservation in early breast cancer. *Int J Radiat Oncol Biol Phys* 13:1327–1332.

NIH Consensus Conference. (1991) Treatment of early-stage breast cancer. *J Natl Cancer Inst: Monographs* (1992) 11:1–5.

Olivotto IA, Rose MA, Osteen RT, et al. (1989) Late cosmetic outcome after conservative surgery and radiotherapy: Analysis of causes of cosmetic failure. *Int J Radiat Oncol Biol Phys* 17:747–753.

Recht A, Siddon RL, Kaplan WD, Andersen JW, Harris JR. (1988) Three-dimensional internal mammary lymphoscintigraphy: Implications for radiation therapy treatment planning for breast carcinoma. *Int J Radiat Oncol Biol Phys* 14:477–481.

Recht A, Harris JR. (1990) Selection of patients with early-stage breast cancer for conservative surgery and radiation. *Oncology* 4:23–30.

Recht A, Pierce SM, Abner A, et al. (1991) Regional nodal failure after conservative surgery and radiotherapy for early stage breast carcinoma. *J Clin Oncol* 9:988–996.

Schmidt–Ullrich R, Wazer DE, Tercilla O, et al. (1989) Tumor margin assessment as a guide to optimal conservation surgery and irradiation in early stage breast carcinoma. *Int J Radiat Oncol Biol Phys* 17:733-738.

Solin LJ, Fowble BL, Schultz DJ, Goodman RL. (1991) The significance of the pathology margins of the tumor excision on the outcome of patients treated with definitive irradiation for early stage breast cancer. *Int J Radiat Oncol Biol Phys* 21:279–287.

Straus K, Lichter A, Lippman M, et al. (1992) Results of the National Cancer Institute early breast cancer trial. *J Natl Cancer Inst Monogr* 11:27–32.

Triedman SA, Osteen R, Harris JR.(1990) Factors influencing cosmetic outcome of conservative surgery and radiotherapy for breast cancer. *Surg Clin North Am* 70:901–916.

van Dongen JA, Bartelink H, Fentiman IS, et al. (1992) Randomized clinical trial to assess the value of breast-conserving therapy in Stage I and II breast cancer, EORTC 10801 trial. *J Natl Cancer Inst Monogr* 11:15–18.

Vicini F, Recht A, Abner A, Silver B, Harris JR. (1990) The association between very young age and recurrence in the breast in pts treated with conservative surgery (CS) and radiation therapy (RT) (abstr). *Int J Radiat Oncol Biol Phys* 19 (suppl 1):132.

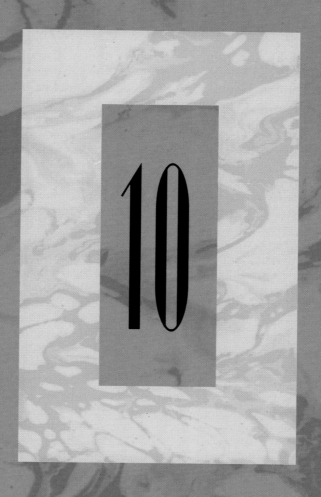

Principles of
Systemic Therapy

Daniel F. Hayes

dentification of risk factors and the use of screening mammography are designed to detect breast cancer while it is still confined to the breast. However, in a substantial number of patients the cancer has already spread beyond the confines of the breast and metastasized to other organs by the time the original breast primary is detected. Therefore, although local therapy is important, diagnosis and therapy of metastatic breast cancer are also critical for patients with this disease. Of the common solid tumors, breast cancer is one of the most responsive to systemic therapy. Two types of systemic modalities are effective in the treatment of breast cancer: chemotherapy, which consists of agents that are specifically cytotoxic; and hormone therapy, which involves using agents or modalities that alter the endocrine milieu and therefore affect tumor cell growth. Chemotherapy and endocrine therapy effectively prevent relapse and prolong the survival of patients with newly diagnosed primary cancer who have evidence of micrometastases but who have no grossly detectable recurrence. This is called adjuvant systemic therapy (see Chapter 11). In patients who have grossly detectable metastatic disease, the agents are used to improve quality of life by reducing symptoms as a result of shrinkage of the tumor masses (see Chapter 12).

CHEMOTHERAPY

Chemotherapeutic agents interfere with essential cell processes, leading to cell death (Fig. 10.1). Although many agents have pleiotropic mechanisms of action (meaning that one agent has several different mechanisms), efforts have been made to classify chemotherapeutic agents according to their presumed primary mechanism of action. Some agents interfere with DNA replication. One process by which this occurs is through the alkylation of base pairs of the cellular DNA, which causes the strands of DNA to form cross-linkages. A second is through intercalation of the drug into the double helix structure of DNA. Both of these mechanisms disrupt normal DNA replication and/or

transcription. Cytotoxic agents may also serve as analogues of substrates of enzymes required for DNA replication and/or transcription. These agents are called antimetabolites. Cytotoxicity also occurs through interference with the normal function of required cellular cytoplasmic or membrane proteins. For example, some agents disrupt the integrity of the cell membrane and prevent normal cellular homeostasis. The vinca alkaloids disturb the normal cellular microtubular function by preventing polymerization of dimers into microtubules and therefore disrupt mitosis. On the other hand, new anticancer agents such as the taxoids (e.g. docetaxel) disrupt mitosis by preventing depolymerization of microtubules into tubulin. None of these agents is specific for cancer cells, and therefore all are toxic to normal cells as well. However, most of these agents work only when cells are in the active stages of the cell cycle (Fig. 10.2). The therapeutic-to-toxic ratio for chemotherapeutic drugs is provided principally by virtue of the higher cell turnover rate associated with neoplastic cells. As a result, the most frequently associated side effects of chemotherapy are seen in normal organs with high cellular growth fractions: suppression of bone marrow and gastrointestinal mucosal function, and hair loss.

Not all chemotherapeutic agents are active against every type of tumor. The most active, and therefore most commonly used, chemotherapeutic drugs for breast cancer include the alkylating agents (cyclophosphamide, L-phenylalanine mustard, thiotepa), the anthracyclines (doxorubicin), the antimetabolites (methotrexate, 5-fluorouracil), the taxoids (e.g. docetaxel) and certain vinca alkaloids (vinblastine) (Fig. 10.3).

HORMONE THERAPY

Many breast cancer cells are also sensitive to hormone therapy. As noted in Chapter 3, normal breast epithelial tissue is organized into lobules, which are composed of clusters of acini and ductules. Breast growth and development appear to depend on a complicated set of interactions among hormones and growth factors

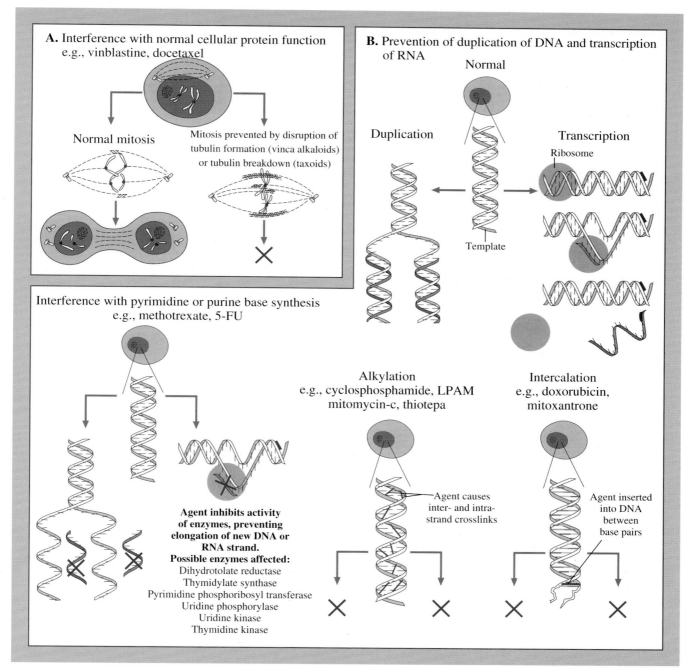

A. Interference with normal cellular protein function
e.g., vinblastine, docetaxel

Normal mitosis

Mitosis prevented by disruption of tubulin formation (vinca alkaloids) or tubulin breakdown (taxoids)

B. Prevention of duplication of DNA and transcription of RNA

Normal

Duplication

Transcription

Ribosome

Template

Interference with pyrimidine or purine base synthesis
e.g., methotrexate, 5-FU

**Agent inhibits activity of enzymes, preventing elongation of new DNA or RNA strand.
Possible enzymes affected:**
Dihydrotolate reductase
Thymidylate synthase
Pyrimidine phosphoribosyl transferase
Uridine phosphorylase
Uridine kinase
Thymidine kinase

Alkylation
e.g., cyclosphosphamide, LPAM mitomycin-c, thiotepa

Agent causes inter- and intra-strand crosslinks

Intercalation
e.g., doxorubicin, mitoxantrone

Agent inserted into DNA between base pairs

Figure 10.1 Possible sites and mechanisms of action of chemotherapeutic agents. In preparation for mitosis, cells duplicate their content of DNA. This process requires synthesis of new purine and pyrimidine bases through a series of enzymatic steps. To maintain normal homeostasis, the genetic code is transcribed, resulting in strands of m-RNA which are translated into proteins. These proteins are responsible for normal structural and functional activities. Chemotherapeutic agents interfere with one or more of these cellular processes. Commonly used chemotherapeutic agents against breast cancer include: alkylating agents, which induce cross-linkages between and within DNA strands; anthracyclines, which intercalate within DNA complexes; antimetabolites, which prevent purine and pyrimidine synthesis; and agents that bind to normal cell proteins such as vinca alkaloids (e.g., vinblastine) and taxoids (e.g. docetaxel).

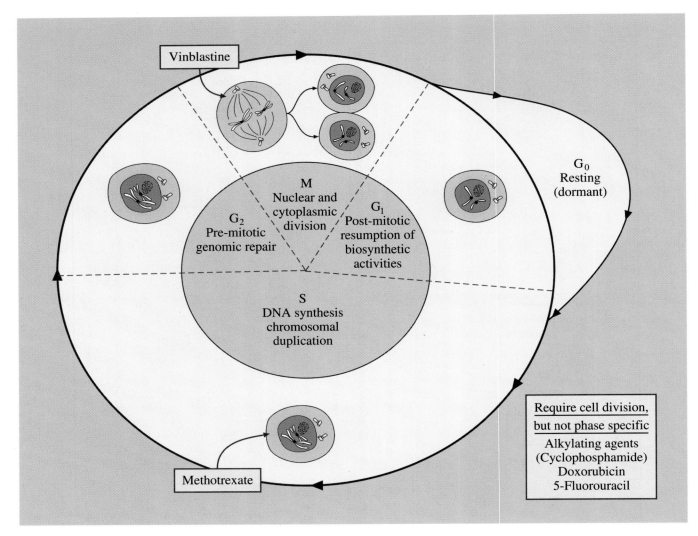

Figure 10.2 Cell cycle. Dividing cells proceed through a series of stages in a cyclic fashion. A large fraction of cells in any given population are in the G_0 stage (resting or dormant). They next enter the cell cycle in G_1, when biosynthetic activity is resumed. In S-phase, new DNA is synthesized and chromosomes are duplicated. In G_2 phase, any errors that occurred during DNA synthesis are repaired and the cell is prepared for mitosis. In M-phase, nuclear and cytoplasmic organelles are replicated, and one cell becomes two. The cell then re-enters G_1 or G_0. Certain chemotherapeutic agents appear to be most effective in particular stages of the cell cycle, although others are relatively cell-cycle independent.

that may be secreted both by the cell itself, by surrounding cells, or by cells at distant sites (autocrine, paracrine, endocrine, respectively) (Fig. 10.4). These hormones and growth factors appear to control breast cell growth and homeostasis by interacting with specific cellular hormone receptors. Two types of hormones influence breast cancer cells: polypeptides and steroids. Recent studies have demonstrated that certain polypeptide hormones specifically interact with cell surface receptors, which then transduce signals intracellularly to the nucleus. These hormones have both stimulatory and inhibitory effects on cell growth. At present, no therapies exist that exploit these polypeptide growth hormone–receptor systems, although it is anticipated that such therapies will become available in the future.

Normal breast epithelial cells and their malignant counterparts are also very sensitive to the effects of steroid hormones, specifically estrogens, progesterones, and androgens. These effects are mediated through steroid hormone receptors, the most well known of which are the estrogen receptor protein and progesterone receptor protein (see Fig. 10.4). Estrogen primarily appears to stimulate normal ductal growth, whereas progesterone is responsible for lobulo-alveolar development. These lipid-soluble molecules diffuse easily through the cell membrane and bind to cytoplasmic receptors, which are then transported to the nucleus where they interact with DNA. This interaction then stimulates appropriate genetic responses that dictate normal cellular growth and "housekeeping" functions.

Figure 10.3 Active Chemotherapeutic Agents in Breast Cancer

Class	Agents
Alkylating Agents	Cyclophosphamide L-Phenylaline Mustard (LPAM) Thiotepa Mitomycin-C
Intercalators (Anthracyclines, anthraquinones)	Doxorubicin Mitoxantrone
Antimetabolites	Methotrexate 5-Fluorouracil
Antitubulins	Vinblastine

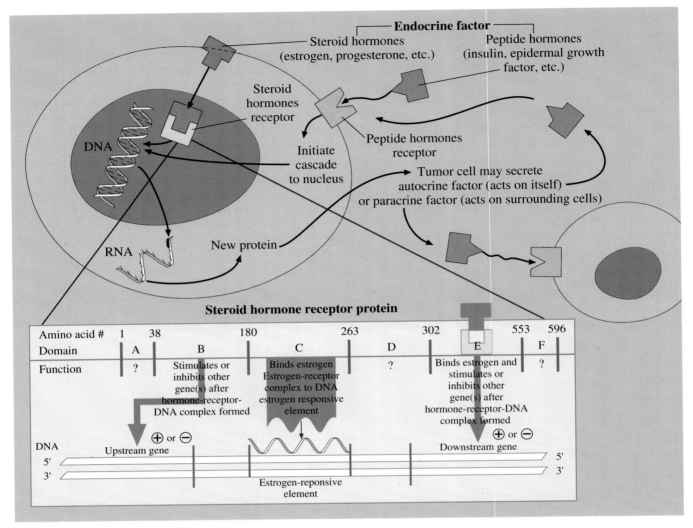

Figure 10.4 Hormonal control of breast cancer cells. These cells are under the control of both steroid hormones and peptide hormones, which can be endocrine (secreted by cells at distant sites), paracrine (secreted by neighboring cells in the immediate area), or autocrine (secreted by the cell itself). Steroid hormones such as estrogen and progesterone freely diffuse through the cell membrane and interact with a cytoplasmic–nuclear receptor. The hormone–receptor complex then binds to DNA and regulates tran-

scription of other genes. Peptide hormones such as insulin, epidermal growth factor, and transforming growth factor bind to cell surface receptors to stimulate conformational changes, with subsequent activation of protein kinases and protein phosphatases. These actions initiate a cascade of signal transductions that ultimately results in stimulation or inhibition of other genes at the DNA level.

A certain fraction of breast cancers express estrogen (ER) and progesterone receptor (PR) proteins, and cell growth and viability appear to be hormone dependent. However, expression of ER and PR is not universal, and the probability that a given tumor will be ER positive is age dependent, although the same may not be true for PR content (Fig. 10.5). Furthermore, breast cancers taken from different sites within the same patient may have different ER contents, and immunohistochemical studies have even demonstrated cell–cell heterogeneity within the same tumor specimen (Fig. 10.6).

Estrogen and progesterone receptor content is measured in several different ways (see Chapter 6). Knowledge of the ER content of a breast cancer is important for two reasons. Tumors with high ER or PR content are better differentiated, and patients with these tumors have a better prognosis (see below). In addition, tumor concentration of ER and PR protein is strongly predictive of response to endocrine therapy (Fig. 10.7).

The mechanisms of action of hormone therapy have not been fully elucidated. However, it is generally believed that manipulation of the hormonal environ-

Figure 10.5 Estrogen and Progesterone Receptor Content According to Patient Age

Age	ER+ (%)	Median ER	PR+ (%)	Median PR
<50	62	8	53	6
>50	80	44	54	6

(From Clark, Osborne, and McGuire, 1984.)

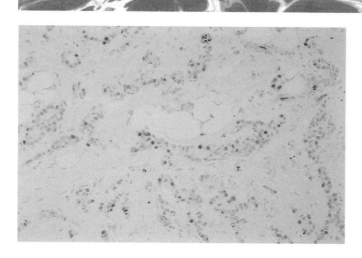

Figure 10.6 Heterogeneity of estrogen receptor. Breast cancer tissue has been evaluated for the presence of ER by immunoperoxidase staining with monoclonal antibodies against the receptor. Even within this single microscopic field, it can be seen that some cells are strongly positive (brown nuclei) whereas other cells are not (blue nuclei). This illustrates the heterogeneity of breast cancer cells.

ment influences division and viability of steroid hormone-dependent breast cancer cells. Several different hormone therapies have been used (Fig. 10.8). The effects of these therapies appear to be a result either of elimination of estrogen production (oophorectomy, progestin therapy, aminoglutethimide, LHRH analogues, adrenalectomy, hypophysectomy) or of blockade of estrogen effects at the cellular level (tamoxifen). Some agents may exert a negative effect on the cell itself (estrogens, androgens, ?progestins, ?tamoxifen).

MECHANISMS OF RESISTANCE

Although it is not entirely clear how all systemic therapies produce their beneficial effects, various mechanisms of resistance have been elucidated (Fig. 10.9) and several different clinical strategies have been developed to attempt to overcome these mechanisms of resistance. It appears that for each course of chemotherapy a constant logarithmic fraction of cells is killed (Fig. 10.10). This theory would explain why most agents have some form of dose response, since an

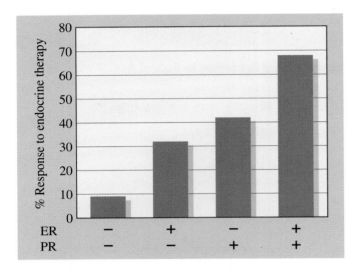

Figure 10.7 Response to endocrine therapy based on estrogen and progesterone receptor content. (Adapted from Clark, Osborne, and McGuire, 1984.)

Figure 10.8 Endocrine Therapies Used in Breast Cancer

Type	Specific Modality Agent
Surgical ablation	Oophorectomy Adrenalectomy Hypophysectomy
Estrogen	Diethylstilbestrol
Androgens	Fluoxymestrone
Antiestrogen	Tamoxifen
Progestins	Megestrol acetate Medroxyprogesterone acetate
Hydroxylase/aromatase inhibitor	Aminoglutethamide
LHRH analogues	Leuprolide

Figure 10.9 Possible Mechanisms of Resistance to Chemotherapy

Pharmacologic sanctuaries (e.g., brain, testis)

Decreased transmembrane transport of drug into cell (influx)

Decreased intracellular activation of drug

Decreased sensitivity of target proteins to effects of drug

  Gene amplification

  Alternate pathways

  Altered pools of substrates

  Altered target (e.g., enzymes, tubular proteins)

Increased repair of damaged DNA

Increased intracellular metabolism of drug

Increased transmembrane transport of drug from cell (efflux)

increase in dose might increase the number of logarithms of cells killed per course of therapy. Clinically, optimal doses are determined to deliver maximum concentrations to the cell. Combination chemotherapy attacks cancer cells with multiple drugs that work by several different mechanisms, thus making resistance to a single agent less important (Fig. 10.11). Most chemotherapeutic agents are given in combination at maximally tolerated doses. In breast cancer, the most commonly used regimens are cyclophosphamide, methotrexate, and 5-fluorouracil (CMF) and cyclophosphamide, doxorubicin (Adriamycin), and 5-fluorouracil (CAF). The benefits of combination, high-dose hormone therapy have not been demonstrated, possibly because endocrine treatment may function through mechanisms distinct from those of chemotherapy.

TOXICITY

As previously noted, systemic therapy, especially chemotherapy, is not without toxicity. Since chemotherapy principally affects rapidly dividing cells, the most common side effects of most chemotherapeutic agents include nausea, vomiting, hair loss, gastrointestinal symptoms (diarrhea and mucosal ulcerations), and bone marrow depression. These side effects vary in intensity according to the specific drug used and to its dose and the method of administration. In addition, each of the specific agents also has one or more relatively unique side effects that must be considered. For example, cyclophosphamide may cause urinary cystic hemorrhage, which can be prevented by adequate hydration. Doxorubicin is associated with an increased incidence of heart failure when given at cumulative doses above 400–450 mg/M2 over a patient's lifetime.

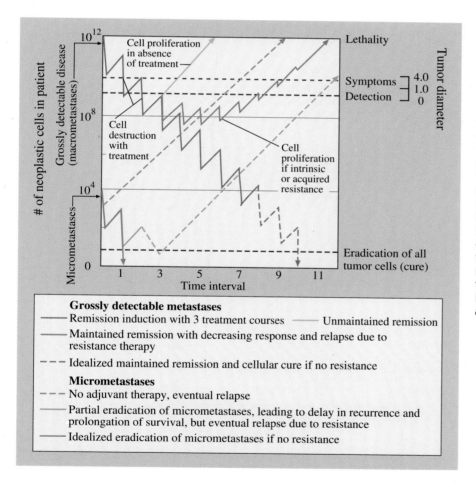

Grossly detectable metastases
—— Remission induction with 3 treatment courses   —— Unmaintained remission
—— Maintained remission with decreasing response and relapse due to resistance therapy
– – – Idealized maintained remission and cellular cure if no resistance
Micrometastases
– – – No adjuvant therapy, eventual relapse
—— Partial eradication of micrometastases, leading to delay in recurrence and prolongation of survival, but eventual relapse due to resistance
—— Idealized eradication of micrometastases if no resistance

Figure 10.10 Theoretical logarithmic killing of neoplastic cells by chemotherapy. For each course of chemotherapy a constant logarithmic fraction of malignant cells is killed. Several theoretical possibilities may occur. The tumor may be sensitive to the agents used, and continued treatment with these agents may lead to eradication of the tumor. The tumor may be sensitive for a brief period of time but ultimately resistant cells become dominant and the tumor grows. In patients with micrometastases, the same or perhaps greater logarithmic cell kill occurs as in patients with macrometastases, except that in this model fewer cells are present at the initiation of chemotherapy, as might be expected in the case of adjuvant chemotherapy for micrometastases. Furthermore, the cells in the micrometastatic setting may also be less resistant. (Modified from Bloom, Frei, and Holland, 1982, with permission.)

5-Fluorouracil may cause cerebellar dysfunction in an occasional patient. In addition to damage to gastrointestinal mucosa, methotrexate may also cause renal and hepatic toxicity, although this is unusual at conventional doses. A few patients have been reported to be allergic to methotrexate, having manifested both dermal and pulmonary reactions.

In general, endocrine therapy has a much lower incidence of side effects than chemotherapy. Tamoxifen is usually quite well tolerated for long periods of time. Of interest is that tamoxifen has weak estrogenic activity in nonmammary tissues. This characteristic might actually protect against osteoporosis and premature coronary artery disease at the same time that it prevents breast cancer recurrence. However, these observations are preliminary and have been made only in postmenopausal women. Ongoing studies should further delineate the long-term benefits and toxicities of tamoxifen. Other side effects of hormone therapies are listed in Figure 10.12.

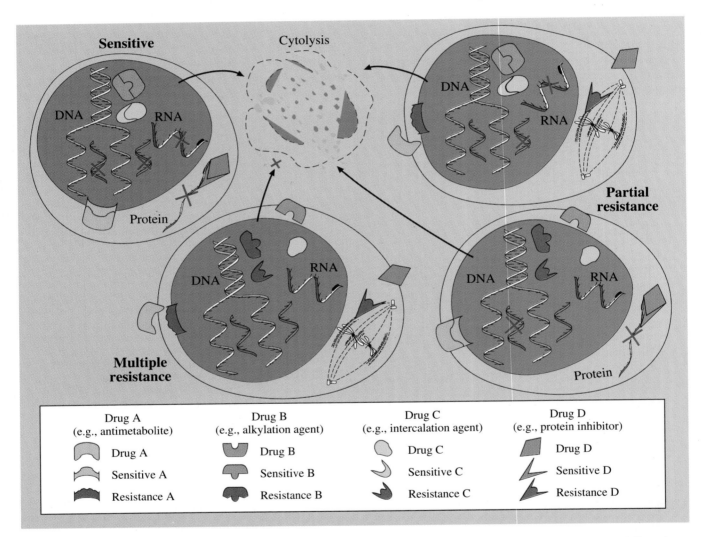

Figure 10.11 Combination chemotherapy. Cells within a single tumor may develop multiple mechanisms of resistance to different chemotherapeutic agents. Therefore, treatment with a single drug might be less effective than treatment with multiple drugs, since the latter interferes with cellular function at several different sites. In the sensitive cell, all four drugs (A–D) are effective. In these cells single-agent chemotherapy would be expected to be as effective as combination chemotherapy. In the partially resistant cells, resistance has developed to one or more of the agents. In this case, combination chemotherapy would be expected to kill both cells, although by different mechanisms. Cells with multiple resistance are not sensitive to any of the chemotherapeutic agents. This type of resistance results in continued cell growth despite chemotherapy, and ultimate mortality.

Figure 10.12 Common Toxicities of Hormone Therapies

Modality/Agent	Common Side Effects (More than 1% of Patients May Experience)
Oophorectomy	Menopausal symptoms (hot flashes, etc.) Osteoporosis Increased risk for coronary artery disease
Adrenolectomy	Addison's syndrome
Hypophysectomy	Panhypopituitarism

Diethylstilbestrol	Gynecologic symptoms
	    Nipple pigmentation
	    Breast engorgement
	    Breast tenderness
	    Vaginal bleeding
	Gastrointestinal symptoms
	Edema
	Incontinence
	Congestive heart failure

Fluoxymestrone	Masculinization Gastrointestinal symptoms Edema Hypercalcemia

Tamoxifen	Gastrointestinal symptoms
	Gynecologic symptoms
	    Menopausal symptoms
	    Vaginal discharge
	    Vaginal bleeding
	Rash
	Headache
	Thrombophlebitis
	Hypercalcemia (flare)

Megestrol acetate, medroxyprogesterone acetate	Gynecologic symptoms Gastrointestinal symptoms Weight gain Cushing syndrome Fluid retention Hypertension Acne Diabetes mellitus Rash
Aminoglutethamide	Lethargy Dizziness Ataxia Rash Gastrointestinal symptoms
Leuprolide	Menopausal symptoms

SUGGESTED READING

Blum RH, Frei III E, Holland JF. (1982) Principles of dose, schedule, and combination chemotherapy. In: Holland JF, Frei E III, eds. *Cancer Medicine*. Philadelphia: Lea & Febinger, 730–752.

Chabner B, Collins J. (1990) *Cancer Chemotherapy: Principles and Practice*. Philadelphia: JB Lippincott.

Clark G, Osborne C, McGuire W. (1984) Correlations between estrogen receptor, progesterone receptor, and patient characteristics in human breast cancer. *J Clin Oncol* 2:1102–1109.

DeVita V. (1983) The relationship between tumor mass and resistance to chemotherapy: implication for surgical adjuvant treatment of cancer. *Cancer* 51:1209–1220.

Devita VT. (1989) Principles of chemotherapy. In: DeVita V, Hellman S, Rosenberg S, eds. *Principles and Practice of Oncology*, 3rd ed. Philadelphia: JB Lippincott, 276–300.

Goldie J, Coldman A. (1979) A mathematic model for relating the drug sensitivity of tumors to their spontaneous mutation rate. *Cancer Treat Rep* 63:1727–1733.

Goldie J, Coldman A. (1983) Quantitative model for multiple levels of drug resistance in clinical tumors. *Cancer Treat Rep* 67:923–931.

Henderson IC. (1991) Chemotherapy for metastatic breast cancer. In: Harris JR, Hellman S, Henderson IC, Kinne DW, eds. *Breast Diseases*, 2nd ed. Philadelphia: JB Lippincott, 604–665.

Henderson IC. (1991) Endocrine therapy of metastatic breast cancer. In: Harris JR, Hellman S, Henderson IC, Kinne DW, eds. *Breast Diseases*, 2nd ed. Philadelphia: JB Lippincott, 559–603.

Osborne CK. (1991) Receptors. In: Harris J, Hellman S, Henderson IC, Kinne DW, eds. *Breast Diseases*, 2nd ed. Philadelphia: JB Lippincott, 301–325.

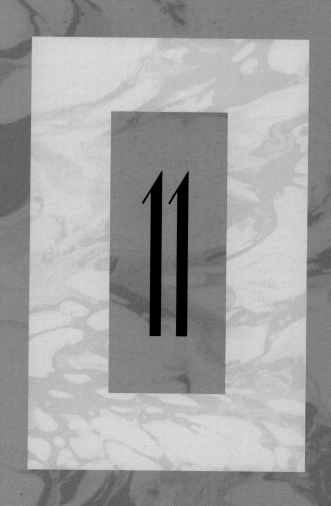

11

Adjuvant Systemic Therapy

Daniel F. Hayes

Patients with grossly detectable metastatic disease often respond to hormone therapy or chemotherapy and may benefit from a reduction in their tumor-related symptoms. However, these patients are rarely, if ever, cured of their disease. Animal models studied in the 1960s and 1970s suggested that resistance might develop as a function of genetic instability that occurred during multiple mitoses and expansion of the tumor cell line (Fig. 11.1). These studies led to investigation of the delivery of systemic therapy at a time when patients were clinically free of disease but were felt to be at high risk for distant recurrence. (In other words, they are very likely to have residual micrometastases; see Chapter 1.) The administration of either hormone therapy or chemotherapy (or performance of an oophorectomy) to patients who do not have grossly detectable metastatic disease has been termed *adjuvant therapy*. Multiple large

randomized trials have now demonstrated that for most patients who are at risk for recurrence, administration of adjuvant systemic therapy is more effective than giving therapy at the time of clinically documented relapse (Early Breast Cancer Trialists' Collaborative Group, 1992). These studies demonstrate that not only is the time to eventual relapse delayed with the use of adjuvant systemic therapy but that patients who receive adjuvant systemic therapy are also less likely to die of breast cancer than those who do not receive adjuvant therapy (Figs. 11.2 and 11.3).

Despite the widespread acceptance of adjuvant systemic therapy for breast cancer, the benefits of adjuvant systemic therapy are not always easy to relate, either to physicians or patients. Often these benefits are expressed as the absolute difference in either relapse-free survival or overall survival at a given timepoint for

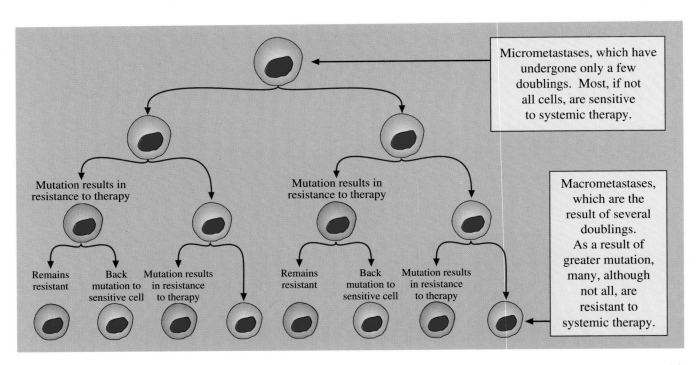

Figure 11.1 Development of increased resistance with cell growth. When a tumor is in its micrometastatic stage, more cells are expected to be in the cell cycle and not in G_0. Therefore, more cells are exposed to the lethal effects of cytotoxic chemotherapy (see Fig. 10.2). Furthermore, because of the genetic instability of tumor cells, mutations occur with subsequent mitoses that provide resistance to chemotherapeutic agents. Therefore, a tumor mass would be expected to be more sensitive when it is smaller and micrometastatic than when it is larger and grossly detectable.

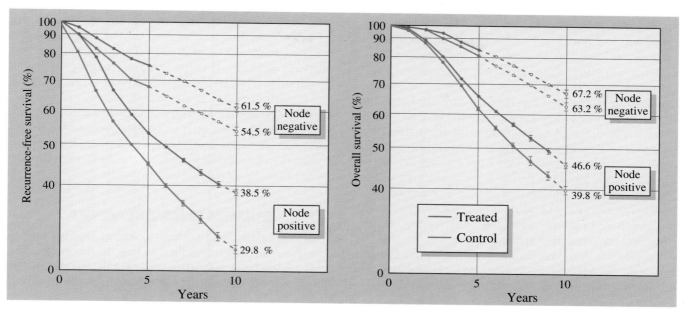

Figure 11.2 Results of overview analysis of adjuvant chemotherapy. Adjuvant chemotherapy reduces the odds of recurrence and mortality in patients with Stage I and II breast cancer, as can be seen in an overview analysis of all randomized studies of adjuvant therapy. Combination chemotherapy results in a highly statistically significant improvement in both of these endpoints (recurrence, mortality) in both node-negative patients and node-positive patients. These results are at 10 years of follow-up. (Modified from Early Breast Cancer Trialists' Collaborative Group, 1992, with permission.)

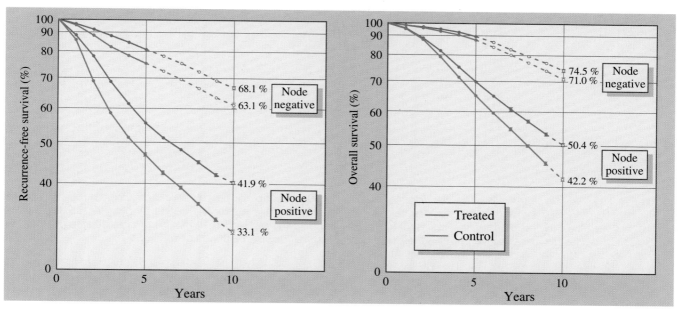

Figure 11.3 Results of overview analysis of adjuvant tamoxifen therapy. As in Figure 11.2, these curves demonstrate that tamoxifen is also highly likely to reduce the odds of recurrence or mortality due to breast cancer in patients with either node-negative or node-positive disease. The effects of either chemotherapy or tamoxifen on specific subgroups of patients (pre- versus postmenopausal, ER-positive versus ER-negative patients) remains controversial. These results are at 10 years. (Modified from Early Breast Cancer Trialists' Collaborative Group, 1992, with permission.)

those patients who received adjuvant therapy versus those who did not (Fig. 11.4A). However, this approach erroneously suggests that only a small percentage of patients benefitted from the therapy. A more meaningful interpretation of the same curves can be made by comparing the median survival time of the treated group with that of the control group. In this way the average difference in survival time for the entire population can be determined (Fig. 11.4B). Although some patients will not achieve this benefit, and others will achieve much longer benefits, a discussion of the average prolongation of survival with a patient about to receive therapy may be more meaningful to her than a discussion of absolute percentage differences between two curves at some arbitrary time point.

Another way of discussing the benefits of adjuvant systemic therapy is to define the relative benefits rather than the absolute benefits for any given popula-

tion. In this case, one must define the absolute risk of the event's occurring (relapse or death). In general, the *relative* reduction in the absolute risk produced by adjuvant systemic therapy remains roughly the same for patients who are at high or low *absolute* risk (Fig. 11.5). Although this is a powerful method of expressing benefits, it must be remembered that this approach demonstrates benefit only in those patients who would suffer recurrence or death from the disease. It essentially ignores the toxicity that all patients experience, even if they never recur.

ASSESSING PROGNOSTIC FACTORS

If adjuvant therapy provides a constant relative reduction in recurrence, regardless of risk, it is beneficial to treat only those patients who are likely to recur. Therefore, the decision about whether to use adjuvant

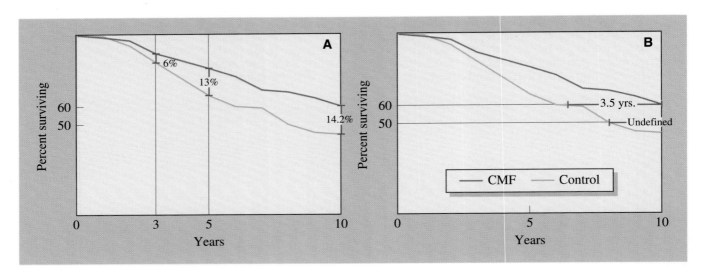

Figure 11.4 Analysis of benefits of adjuvant chemotherapy. (A) The benefits of therapy are expressed in terms of percent differences between the curves at different time points (3, 5, and 10 years). (B) The differences between the curves are expressed in terms of potential prolongation of survival when either 40 percent or 50 percent of the patients have died. One can roughly estimate that the average patient will benefit by between 3.5 and 5 years from having received 6–12 months of chemotherapy. (Modified from Henderson, 1988, with permission.)

systemic therapy depends on two factors: demonstration that the patient is at a reasonably high risk for recurrence and death, and demonstration that the systemic therapy reduces that risk. A number of prognostic factors have been identified to estimate the risk of relapse at the time of primary diagnosis. As noted, patients with proven metastatic disease are rarely if ever cured of their malignancy. Moreover, patients who have locally advanced breast cancer (Stage IIIb) also have very poor prognoses. Fortunately, most patients initially present with Stage I or II breast cancer (see Chapter 1). It is in these patients that prognostic factors are of particular importance (Figure 11.6). The single most important prognostic factor in patients with clinical Stage I or II breast cancer is the presence of histologically involved axillary lymph

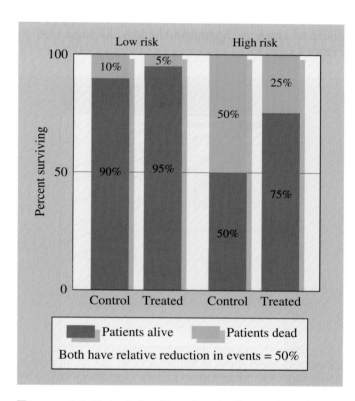

Figure 11.5 Analysis of benefits of adjuvant chemotherapy. This figure illustrates the differences between relative and absolute risk. The bars represent two groups of patients, one with a very low risk of dying of breast cancer (approximately 10 percent) and one with a very high risk of dying of breast cancer (approximately 50 percent). However, the effect of adjuvant systemic therapy in both of these groups is a *relative* reduction in events of approximately 50 percent. In the high-risk group, this reduces the odds of dying from 50 percent to 25 percent (0.5 x 50). Most physicians feel that it is justified to treat the entire population (all of whom will experience side effects) because so many patients are likely to benefit. However, in the low-risk group the reduction of relative risk by 50 percent results in an absolute reduction of only 5 percent (0.5 x 10). Almost 90 percent of the patients who have been treated will not benefit, since they have no risk of relapse. The question of whether these patients should be treated remains highly controversial.

Figure 11.6 Factors That Predict Prognosis in Breast Cancer

Factor	Favorable Association
Size	Small
Palpable lymph nodes	Absent
Pathologic axillary lymph node invasion	Absent
Tissue differentiation	Good
Intratumor lymphatic invasion	Absent
Steroid hormone receptor content	High
Tumor growth rate (S phase fraction)	Low
Miscellaneous	
Cathepsin D content	Low
Her-2/*neu* expression	Low
Tumor neoangiogenesis	Low

SUGGESTED READING

Bonadonna G, Valagussa P. (1989) Systemic therapy in resectable breast cancer. *Hematol Oncol Clin North Am* 3:727–742.

DeVita V. (1983) The relationship between tumor mass and resistance to chemotherapy: implication for surgical adjuvant treatment of cancer. *Cancer* 51:1209–1220.

Early Breast Cancer Trialists' Collaborative Group. (1992) Systemic treatment of early breast cancer by hormonal, cytotoxic, or immune therapy: 133 randomised trials involving 31,000 recurrences and 24,000 deaths among 75,000 women. *Lancet* 2:1–15, 71–85.

Fisher B, Redmond C, Dimitrov N, et al. (1989) A randomized clinical trial evaluating sequential methotrexate and fluorouracil in the treatment of patients with node-negative breast cancer who have estrogen-receptor-negative tumors. *N Engl J Med* 320:473–478.

Fisher B, Constantino J, Redmond C, et al. (1989) A randomized clinical trial evaluating tamoxifen in the treatment of patients with node-negative breast cancer who have estrogen-receptor-positive tumors. *N Engl J Med* 320:479–484.

Fisher B, Redmond C, Wicherham L, et al. (1989) Systemic therapy in patients with node-negative breast cancer: a commentary based on two National Surgical Adjuvant Breast and Bowel Project (NSABP) clinical trials. *Ann Int Med* 111:703–712.

Henderson IC. (1988) Estimating the magnitude of benefits from adjuvant therapy. *Rec Results Cancer Res* 111:82–86.

Henderson IC. (1990) Basic principles in the use of adjuvant therapy. *Semin Oncol* 17:40–44.

Ludwig Breast Cancer Study Group. (1989) Prolonged disease-free survival after one course of perioperative adjuvant chemotherapy for node-negative breast cancer. *N Engl J Med* 320:491–496.

Mansour E, Gray R, Shatila A, et al. (1989) Efficacy of adjuvant chemotherapy in high-risk node-negative breast cancer. *N Engl J Med* 320:485–490.

McGuire W, Meyer J, Barlogie B, et al. (1985) Impact of flow cytometry on predicting recurrence and survival in breast cancer patients. *Breast Cancer Res Treat* 5:117–128.

Nolvadex Adjuvant Trial Organization. (1988) Controlled trial of tamoxifen as single adjuvant agent in management of early breast cancer. *Br J Cancer* 57:608–611.

Osborne CK. (1990) Prognostic factors in breast cancer. *PPO Updates* 4:1–11.

Wilson R, Donegan W, Mettlin C, et al. (1984) The 1982 survey of carcinoma of the breast in the United States by the American College of Surgeons. *Surg Gynecol Obstet* 159:309–318.

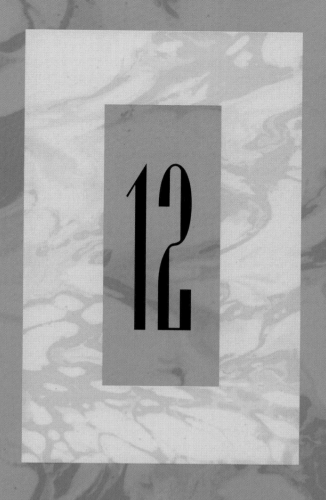

12

Locally Advanced, Locally Recurrent, and Metastatic Breast Cancer

Daniel F. Hayes

Primary and adjuvant systemic therapies for patients with breast cancer are designed to prevent subsequent local and/or distant recurrences. However, approximately one-third of all patients develop locally recurrent and/or metastatic breast cancer. A number of features can help to predict the probability of recurrence or metastasis in newly diagnosed patients (Fig. 12.1). The most important of these factors is clinical stage (see Fig. 12.1). Several studies have suggested that the odds of survival over a five- to ten-year period after initial diagnosis are directly related to clinical stage (Fig. 12.2). Less than 5 percent of patients with newly diagnosed breast cancer present with grossly detectable metastatic disease, which is defined as disease outside of the breast and axillary lymph nodes that can be detected by physical examination or radiographic evaluation. Few if any patients with grossly detectable metastatic disease are cured, even when their disease responds favorably to treatment. Nevertheless, many patients with metastatic disease can live a long time with their disease, which can be palliatively treated by surgery, radiotherapy, hormone therapy, or chemotherapy.

In addition to clinical and radiographic staging, other prognostic factors have been identified (see Fig. 11.1). Of these, the single most important factor is the presence of micrometastasis to axillary lymph nodes (see Fig. 11.6A). As compared with node-negative patients, roughly twice as many node-positive patients suffer distant relapse and mortality over a five- to ten-year period (see Fig. 11.6B). Patients whose tumors are larger also have a slightly worse prognosis. Determination of tumor size can be made quite accurately at the time of specimen processing, as described in Chapter 6. Certain variants of infiltrating ductal carcinoma are associated with a better prognosis, including medullary carcinoma (see Fig. 8.8), mucinous carcinoma (see Fig. 8.9), and tubular carcinoma (see Fig. 8.10). Other histopathologic features may be associated with a worse clinical outcome, including histologic and nuclear differentiation as determined by light microscopy (see Fig. 8.6) and the presence of lymphatic vessel invasion (see Fig. 8.14). The absolute importance of each of these in relation to the presence or absence of other features in the same patient has yet to be determined. Therefore, decisions regarding adjuvant systemic therapy remain difficult and are based principally on clinical and pathologic staging (see Chapter 11).

Locally advanced breast cancer (Stage IIIb) is distinguished by one or more features involving either the primary tumor (T_4) or the regional lymph nodes (N_3) (see Fig. 1.1). The most dramatic of these are clinical inflammation (see Figs. 4.21 and 4.22) and/or skin ulcerations (Fig. 12.3). Patients with Stage III (especially Stage IIIb) disease are at very high risk for subsequent recurrence and mortality, as are patients with local recurrence after mastectomy (see Figs. 4.22, 8.16, 9.24, and 9.25). Many patients with locally advanced breast cancer benefit from a combination of initial (or "proto-adjuvant") systemic therapy followed by local therapy (surgery and/or radiation therapy).

It is important to remember that *no* patient with a prior history of invasive breast cancer is free from the risk of subsequent recurrence. Many patients ultimately die of other diseases without any detectable metastases, and are thus effectively cured. However, throughout the life of a patient who has had invasive breast cancer, the chance exists that she will suffer a distant relapse. For example, relapses have been reported as long as 30 to 40 years after diagnosis, even in patients considered to have good prognoses (Figs. 12.4 and 12.5).

The follow-up management of patients who have been rendered disease-free by primary and adjuvant therapy includes a careful history and physical examination and investigation of symptoms or signs of recurrent cancer, bearing in mind that breast cancer can metastasize to almost any organ or tissue (Fig. 12.6). In addition, certain laboratory tests, including liver function tests and tumor-associated markers, may also indicate the possibility of recurrent disease (Fig. 12.7). Radiographic evaluations, including chest x-rays, bone scans, and more sophisticated analyses with CT and MRI, are helpful in detecting relapse. Finally, specific evaluation of symptomatic or suspected sites with various radiographic tests can be complemented by aspiration or surgical biopsy of tissue for diagnosis.

The clinical value of intensive efforts to detect metastatic breast cancer early is controversial. Early treatment of newly diagnosed primary breast cancer with both local (Chapters 3 and 4) and systemic thera-

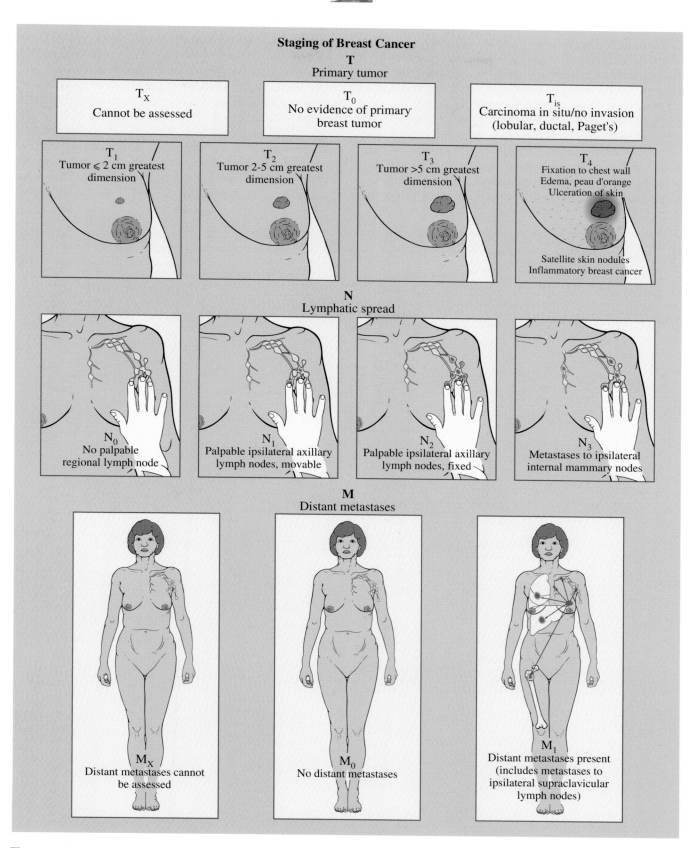

Staging of Breast Cancer

T
Primary tumor

| T_X Cannot be assessed | T_0 No evidence of primary breast tumor | T_{is} Carcinoma in situ/no invasion (lobular, ductal, Paget's) |

T_1
Tumor $\leq$ 2 cm greatest dimension

T_2
Tumor 2-5 cm greatest dimension

T_3
Tumor >5 cm greatest dimension

T_4
Fixation to chest wall
Edema, peau d'orange
Ulceration of skin

Satellite skin nodules
Inflammatory breast cancer

N
Lymphatic spread

N_0
No palpable regional lymph node

N_1
Palpable ipsilateral axillary lymph nodes, movable

N_2
Palpable ipsilateral axillary lymph nodes, fixed

N_3
Metastases to ipsilateral internal mammary nodes

M
Distant metastases

M_X
Distant metastases cannot be assessed

M_0
No distant metastases

M_1
Distant metastases present (includes metastases to ipsilateral supraclavicular lymph nodes)

Figure 12.1 Breast cancer staging, based on clinical characteristics. (From *AJCC*, 1988.)

Locally Advanced, Locally Recurrent, and Metastatic Breast Cancer

py (Chapter 11) has now been shown to be more effective than delayed therapy. However, early treatment of grossly detectable metastatic lesions has not been proven to be more beneficial than treatment of patients with symptomatic disease (Fig. 12.8).

Choosing the appropriate form of therapy for patients with metastatic disease requires careful consideration of the characteristics of the cancer and the goals of both the physician and the patient. For patients with principally local problems, local therapy alone (surgery, radiotherapy) may alleviate symptoms and provide adequate palliation (see Fig. 9.24). In addition, the presence of disease in certain sites such as weight-bearing leg bones or in the spinal canal may cause such severe pain or confer such a high risk of fracture or neurologic dysfunction that local therapy is preferable to systemic therapy. For example, lytic disease involving more than 50 percent of the femoral cortical bone is associated with a high risk of fracture (Fig. 12.9), and breast cancer metastatic to the vertebral column can impinge on the spinal canal and cause spinal cord compression (Figs. 12.10 and 12.11). Both

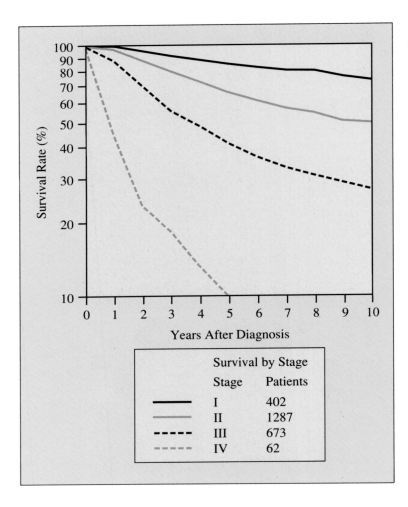

Figure 12.2 Survival of breast cancer patients by stage at the time of diagnosis. The number of patients diagnosed with each stage is also given. (Adapted from Cutler, 1974, with permission.)

Survival by Stage		
	Stage	Patients
———	I	402
———	II	1287
- - - -	III	673
- - - -	IV	62

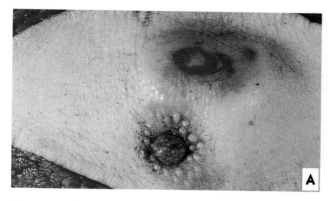

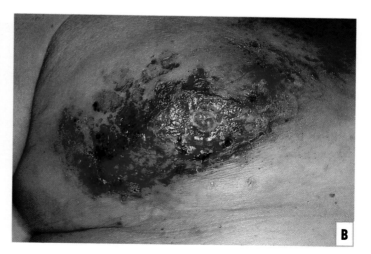

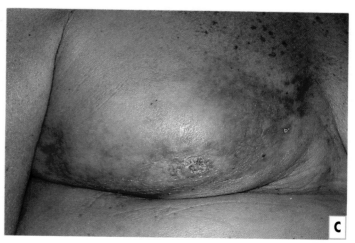

Figure 12.3 Stage IIIB (T$_4$) breast cancer. (A) This patient presented with an ulceration superior to the nipple. An underlying tumor was biopsied and was cytologically diagnosed as infiltrating ductal carcinoma. (B,C) This 66-year-old patient presented with a locally advanced carcinoma that had ulcerated through the skin, causing substantial morbidity (B). She was treated effectively with chemotherapy, and over five months the ulceration decreased and the tumor regressed. Ultimately the skin healed completely (C).

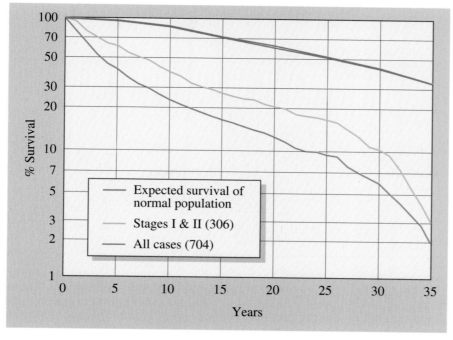

Figure 12.4 Survival curve for breast cancer patients after primary therapy in long-term follow-up. Even as long as 35 years after initial diagnosis and therapy, patients with breast cancer, including those with Stages I and II, continued to relapse and die of their disease. (Modified from Brinkley, Haybittle, and Houghton, 1984, with permission.)

Legend:
— Expected survival of normal population
— Stages I & II (306)
— All cases (704)

Y-axis: % Survival
X-axis: Years

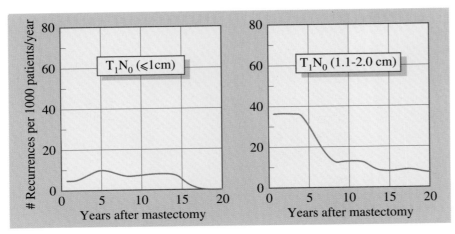

Figure 12.5 Recurrence rates in patients with a good prognosis after long-term follow-up. Even women with good prognoses (T_1N_0, ≤1 cm; T_1N_0 1.1–2.0 cm) suffer recurrences as late as 15 to 20 years after diagnosis. These graphs show the number of women who suffer recurrences during each year of follow-up. (Modified from Rosen, et al., 1989, with permission.)

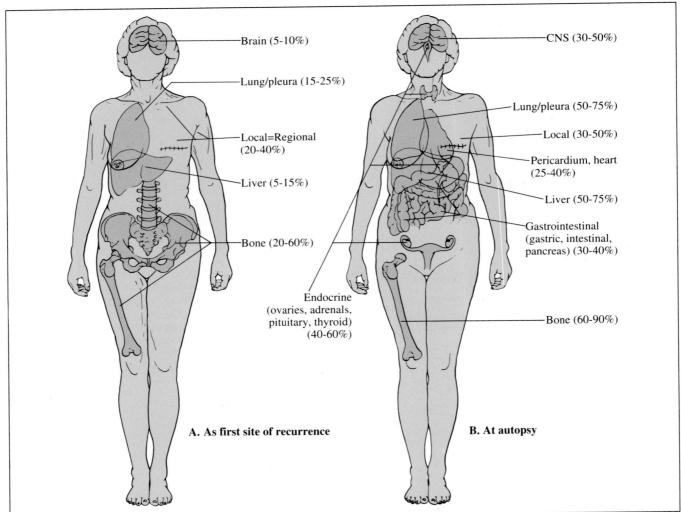

A. As first site of recurrence

B. At autopsy

Figure 12.6 Frequency of breast cancer metastases. (A) The most common first sites of recurrent breast cancer are the chest wall, the regional lymph nodes, and/or the bone. Liver, lung , and central nervous system (CNS) are less common sites of recurrence. (B) In patients with far-advanced disease, breast cancer can be found in almost any organ. Autopsy studies show that metastases are most commonly found in the chest wall and in the surrounding lymph nodes, as well as in the bones, liver, lung, pleura, and CNS (brain, spinal cord, meninges). Metastases may also occur in gastrointestinal organs (pancreas, stomach, large and small intestine), endocrine organs (ovaries, adrenals, pituitary, thyroid), and in the cardiovascular system (pericardium, endocardium, myocardium).

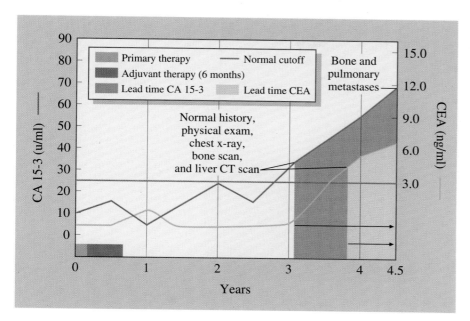

Figure 12.7 Early detection of metastasis with circulating tumor markers. This patient had a Stage II breast cancer treated by breast-conserving therapy and adjuvant chemotherapy. Three years after the completion of all chemotherapy, while the patient was asymptomatic, her serial CA15-3 and CEA levels began to rise. History, physical examination, and radiographic evaluations were all normal. She received no therapy at this time. Approximately one and a half years later she developed bone and pulmonary metastases.

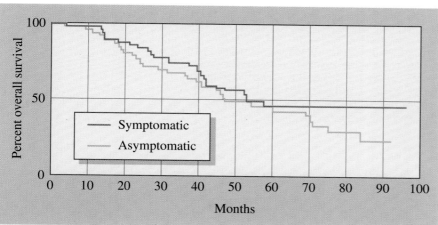

Figure 12.8 Overall survival in patients with metastatic breast cancer, depending on whether patients present with symptomatic or asymptomatic metastasis. In a retrospective study, the overall survival of patients whose metastases were detected and treated before the appearance of symptoms was no better than that for patients whose treatment was delayed until they developed symptoms. (Modified from Stierer and Rosen, 1989, with permission.)

Locally Advanced, Locally Recurrent, and Metastatic Breast Cancer

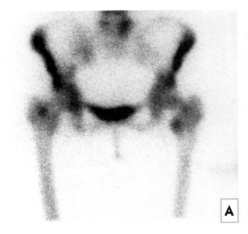

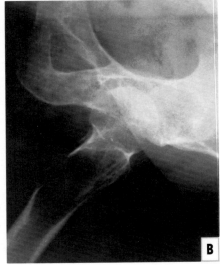

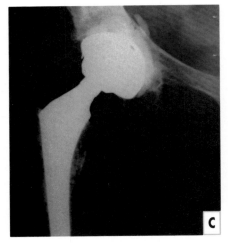

Figure 12.9 Bone metastasis with risk of fracture. Lytic lesions in weight-bearing areas are particularly worrisome. This patient had multiple sites of radionuclide uptake on a bone scan, including the trochanter and the neck of the right femur (A). Plain films of this region demonstrated a very large lytic lesion in the same area that was positive on her bone scan (B). The patient was referred to an orthopedic surgeon and underwent a total right hip replacement, with return of full function. (C) An x-ray of her right hip prosthesis after replacement.

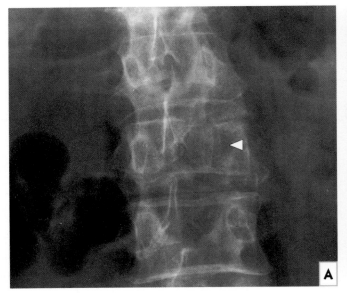

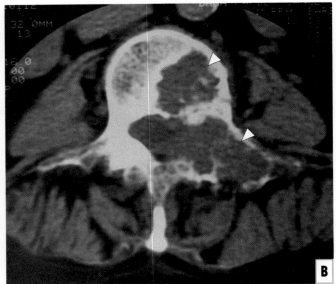

Figure 12.10 Vertebral metastasis with spinal cord compression. (A) Plain film of the lumbar spine demonstrates complete absence of the left pedicle of the L2 vertebra (arrow). (B) On CT scan, a large lytic lesion involves about half of the body of L2, including the left pedicle (arrows). In addition, a soft-tissue mass extends into the spinal canal, compressing the spinal cord. Spinal cord compression is one of the oncologic emergencies that require either immediate decompression or radiation therapy. It can lead to neurologic deficits and even paraplegia. (From Hayes, 1991.)

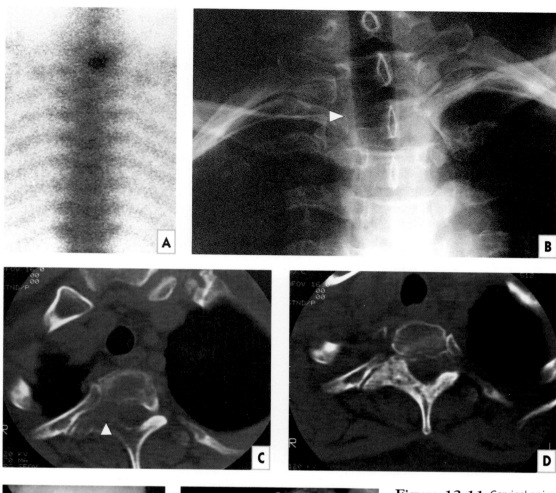

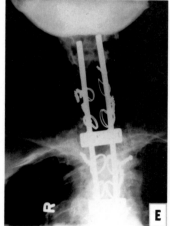

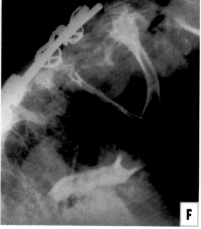

Figure 12.11 Cervical spine metastasis. A common site of metastatic breast cancer is the vertebral column. Although a single area of increased uptake on a bone scan in a long bone may represent a benign process, the same finding in the axial skeleton is highly suspicious for metastatic disease. Metastasis to the cervical spine raises concern about possible spinal cord compression. (A) A patient with a prior history of Stage II breast cancer presented with pain in her upper back, and bone scan demonstrated a single area of uptake on the right side of the T2 vertebral body. Plain radiography revealed an absent right pedicle at T2 (B, *arrow*) corresponding to the same area that was positive on the bone scan. (C) CT scan demonstrated a large lytic lesion (*arrow*) with destruction of the right pedicle. (D) After radiotherapy, a CT scan was performed and demonstrated healing, as determined by sclerosis and recalcification. Unfortunately, this patient subsequently had recurrent progression in this same area. Since she had received the maximal amount of radiation therapy to this region, she was treated surgically. A laminectomy and decompression was performed at T2, and then her cervical spine was stabilized (E,F). These films show the position of the C-spine-stabilizing rods that were placed surgically. The patient recovered and went on to have normal ambulation and use of all extremities.

Locally Advanced, Locally Recurrent, and Metastatic Breast Cancer

of these catastrophic clinical events can be effectively treated or even prevented with surgery, radiotherapy, or both. Similarly, treatment of brain metastasis with radiotherapy frequently achieves satisfactory results, although the long-term prognosis for such patients is poor (Fig. 12.12).

The choice between endocrine therapy and chemotherapy depends on the potential for response and the respective therapy's toxicity (see Chapter 10). However, even allowing for the associated toxicities,

patients often respond well to systemic therapy and experience substantial benefit (Figs. 12.13 to 12.29). The potential toxicity of all forms of systemic therapy (short-term and long-term) must be weighed against the potential benefits (see Chapter 10, Figs. 12.30 to 12.33). Response to therapy is monitored in several ways. If palliation is the goal of therapy, a careful history can be invaluable. Serial physical examinations and measurements of palpable lesions, or serial radiographic and/or scintigraphic evaluations, provide more objec-

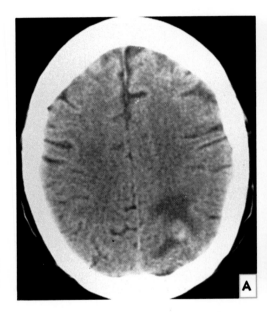
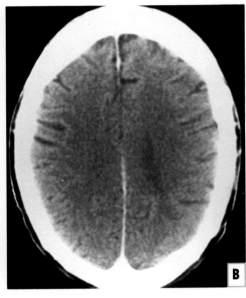

Figure 12.12 Brain metastases. Breast cancer commonly spreads to the brain, causing neurologic morbidity related to the specific site of involvement. Metastases can be single or multiple to the cerebral or cerebellar cortex and/or to the leptomeninges (see Figure 12.20). (A) CT scan of the brain of a 62-year-old woman who presented six years after mastectomy and adjuvant chemotherapy for a Stage II breast carcinoma shows a well-circumscribed enhanc-

ing lesion with surrounding edema in the left temporo–occipital region. She also had pulmonary and hepatic metastases. (B) Repeat CT scan taken three months after completion of successful radiotherapy reveals that the enhancing lesion is no longer evident and the edema has almost completely resolved. Her symptoms also totally resolved. (From Hayes, 1991.)

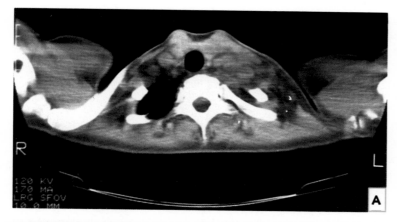

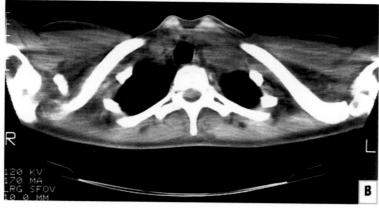

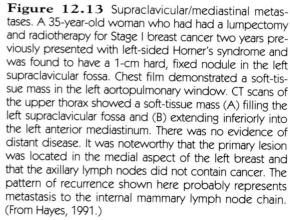

Figure 12.13 Supraclavicular/mediastinal metastases. A 35-year-old woman who had had a lumpectomy and radiotherapy for Stage I breast cancer two years previously presented with left-sided Horner's syndrome and was found to have a 1-cm hard, fixed nodule in the left supraclavicular fossa. Chest film demonstrated a soft-tissue mass in the left aortopulmonary window. CT scans of the upper thorax showed a soft-tissue mass (A) filling the left supraclavicular fossa and (B) extending inferiorly into the left anterior mediastinum. There was no evidence of distant disease. It was noteworthy that the primary lesion was located in the medial aspect of the left breast and that the axillary lymph nodes did not contain cancer. The pattern of recurrence shown here probably represents metastasis to the internal mammary lymph node chain. (From Hayes, 1991.)

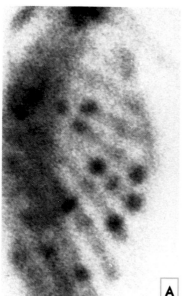

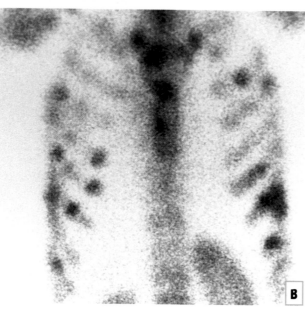

Figure 12.14 Bone metastases. Bone is one of the most common sites of metastatic breast disease. Although benign disorders, such as osteoarthritis, osteomyelitis, or benign fractures, can cause a bone scan to be positive, the appearance of multiple "hot spots," especially in the axial and thoracic skeleton, as shown here (A,B), are highly suggestive of metastases. (From Hayes, 1991.)

Locally Advanced, Locally Recurrent, and Metastatic Breast Cancer

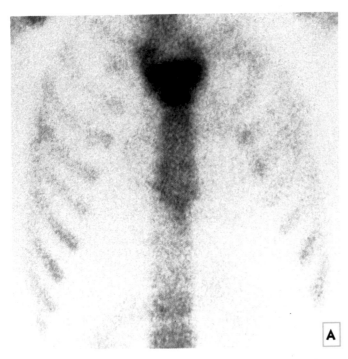

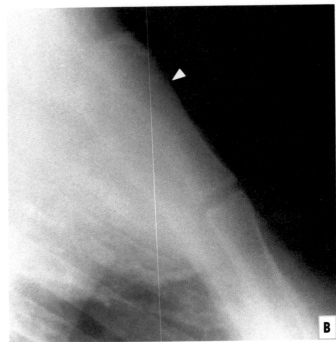

Figure 12.15 Bone metastases. Bone metastases are not always multiple. (A) This bone scan demonstrates an isolated area of increased uptake in the manubrial–sternal area; there was no evidence of other abnormalities. Plain radiographs of suspected areas can help confirm the presence or absence of bone metastases.

Such films may show the presence of a benign lesion, which can explain an abnormal scan. On the other hand, lytic or blastic lesions are suggestive of an underlying carcinoma. (B) Plain film of the sternum reveals a lytic area *(arrow)* corresponding to the "hot spot" on bone scan. (From Hayes, 1991.)

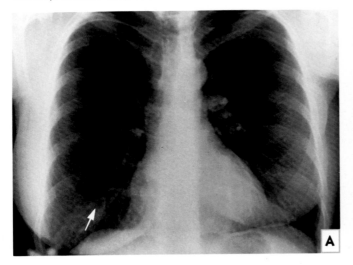

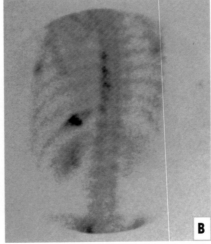

Figure 12.16 Bone metastasis, lytic rib lesion. This 37-year-old woman with Stage II breast cancer was treated with breast-conserving therapy and adjuvant chemotherapy. Three years later she presented with pain in her right lower thoracic wall. A PA chest film was initially read as normal. Closer inspection revealed that a section

of the right eighth rib was absent (A, *arrow*). A subsequent bone scan revealed increased uptake in the right eighth rib in the area corresponding to the chest x-ray findings (B). These radiographs demonstrate the importance of looking not only for the presence of positive findings but also for the absence of normal structures.

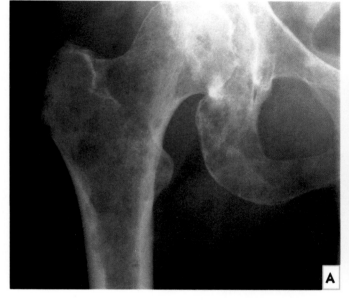

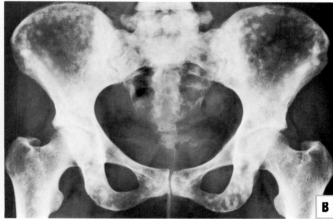

Figure 12.17 Lytic vs. blastic bone metastases. In general, lytic bone metastases are more common than osteoblastic lesions, although many patients exhibit mixed lytic lesions with areas of osteoblastic reaction. (A) Diffuse lytic lesions can be seen in this patient's right femoral head and ischial pubic ramus. Such lesions weaken the cortex, often resulting in pathologic fracture. (B) Radio-graph of the pelvis of a 45-year-old woman demonstrates widespread foci of increased bone density, representing osteoblastic activity surrounding bone metastases of breast cancer. It is interesting to note that effective therapy may alter the nature of lytic bone metastases, converting them to sclerotic, blastic lesions. (From Hayes, 1991.)

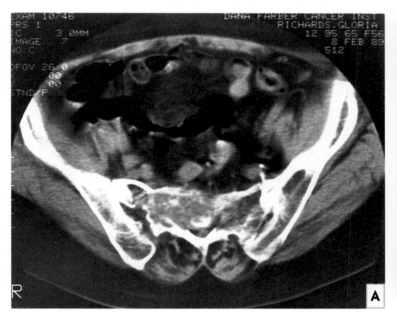

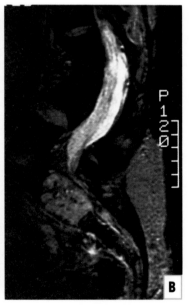

Figure 12.18 Sacral metastases. A postmenopausal woman receiving adjuvant chemotherapy for breast cancer developed pain in her left hip and buttock. Bone scan of the area indicated increased uptake across the left sacroiliac region, and a CT scan (A) revealed bilateral lytic lesions within the sacrum and iliac bones. The tumor appears to extend into the epidural canal and project superiorly toward the lumbar spine. (B) MRI shows that the superior extent of the tumor is well below the end of the spinal cord. As an incidental finding, congenital fusion of her lumbar vertebrae was also noted. Although metastases below L2 or L3 may cause significant symptoms, they do not cause spinal cord compression because these sites are at the level of the cauda equina or sacral nerve roots. (From Hayes, 1991.)

Locally Advanced, Locally Recurrent, and Metastatic Breast Cancer

tive assessments of response. Furthermore, certain circulating tumor markers may serve as helpful adjuncts for predicting a patient's clinical course (Fig. 12.34).

In summary, the primary goal of early detection and treatment of newly diagnosed breast cancer is to reduce morbidity and mortality by preventing metastases and growth in distant organs. The risk of subsequent relapse for a given patient depends on her prognostic factor profile. Any unusual sign or symptom of recurrence should be appropriately evaluated, always considering metastatic breast cancer in the differential diagnosis. Although metastatic breast cancer is rarely curable, it can be effectively treated, providing substantial benefit to the patient in terms of her quality of life, by balancing the potential or actual toxicity of therapy against the reduction in tumor-related symptoms.

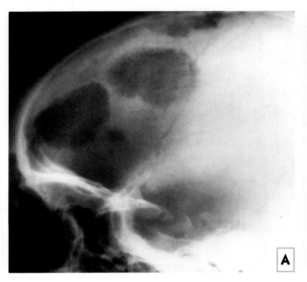 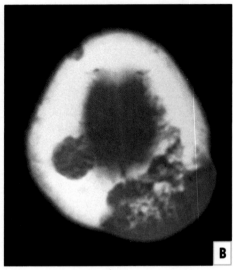

Figure 12.19 Skull metastasis. Breast cancer can metastasize to the skull without involving the brain parenchyma. (A) Plain radiograph demonstrates large lytic metastases in the bones of the cranium. (B) CT scan of another patient with a palpable posterior skull metastasis shows a soft-tissue mass with extension through the thickness of the bone. Although the brain parenchyma was compressed posteriorly, the patient had no neurologic symptoms. (From Hayes, 1991.)

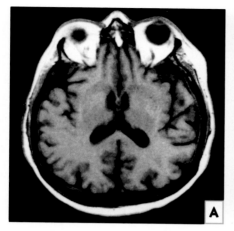

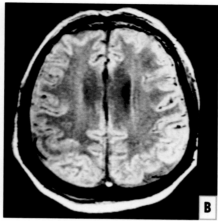

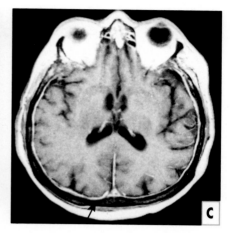

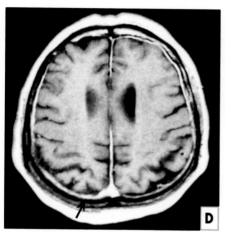

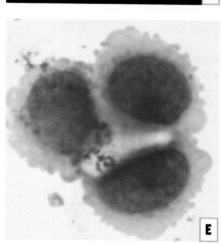

Figure 12.20 Meningeal metastases. In addition to parenchymal CNS metastases (see Fig. 12.14), breast cancer can also spread to the leptomeninges. This 65-year-old woman with known metastatic breast cancer presented with a headache and multiple cranial nerve deficits. MRI without gadolinium was interpreted as normal (A,B). However, with gadolinium enhancement (C,D), the meningeal surface was found to be abnormally thickened *(arrow)*. Lumbar puncture revealed the presence of metastatic breast cancer in the cerebrospinal fluid (E).

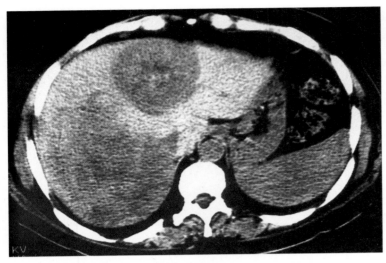

Figure 12.21 Liver metastasis. Liver metastases of breast cancer are usually suspected in the presence of abnormal liver function tests or circulating tumor markers (e.g., CEA or CA15-3). This CT scan demonstrates two very large metastases. (From Hayes, 1991.)

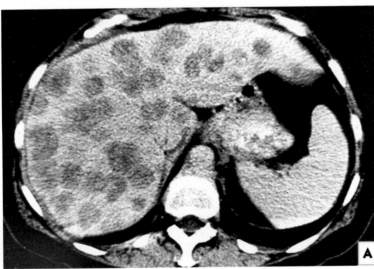

Figure 12.22 Liver metastasis. (A) CT scan of the abdomen in a 40-year-old patient shows multiple discrete lesions within the liver. (B) The response to chemotherapy can be quite impressive. After three courses of chemotherapy, the improvement in the patient's liver is remarkable. (From Hayes, 1991.)

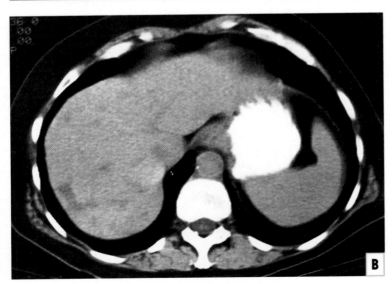

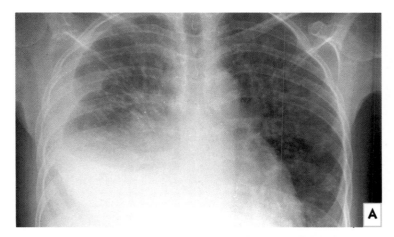

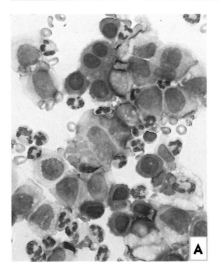

Figure 12.23 Intrathoracic metastases. Intrathoracic metastases can be manifested by several findings. Among the more common is malignant pleural effusion, as demonstrated by the large right effusion on this chest film (A); multiple metastatic pulmonary nodules are also evident. (B) Chest CT scan confirms the pleural effusion; in addition, the advanced right breast cancer can be seen. (From Hayes, 1991.)

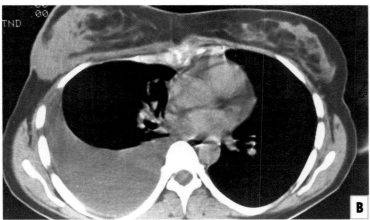

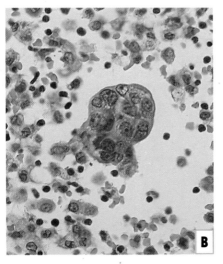

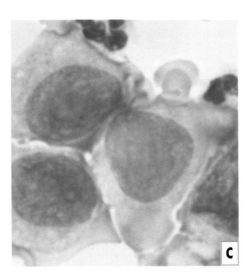

Figure 12.24 Malignant pleural effusion. Pleural effusions are common in patients with breast cancer, resulting from metastatic spread to pleural surfaces or mediastinum. Correct diagnosis may require thoracentesis with biochemical analysis and cytologic examination of the pleural fluid. (A) Low-power view of centrifuge preparation of pleural fluid from a patient with a history of metastatic breast cancer and a new pleural effusion. Large clumps of malignant cells can be seen. (B) Higher-power view of pleural fluid cytologic smear from a second patient showing aggregation of cells with highly pleomorphic cytologic features and distinct nucleoli. The surrounding cells are normal mesothelial cells. (C) High-power view of cytocentrifuge smear of pleural fluid showing a clump of large, bizarre malignant cells with distinct nucleoli. (Fig. 12.26B courtesy of Aron Lukacher, M.D., Brigham and Women's Hospital, Boston, MA.)

Locally Advanced, Locally Recurrent, and Metastatic Breast Cancer

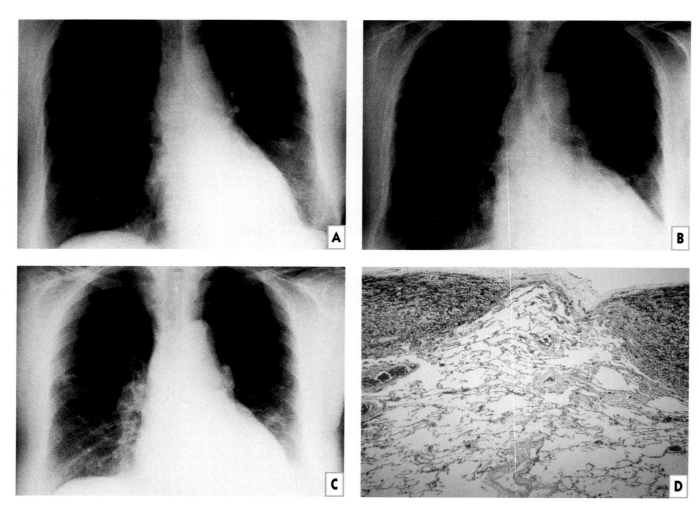

Figure 12.25 Pulmonary nodular metastases. (A) A 63-year-old woman with a prior history of known metastatic disease to bone was found on routine chest x-ray to have asymptomatic pulmonary nodules. (B,C) After hormone therapy with megestrol acetate, the patient's bone pain improved and she was found to have a decrease in the size of her pulmonary nodules. (D) Histopathology of nodular metastasis within normal lung tissue.

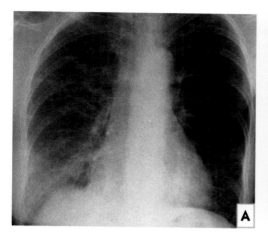

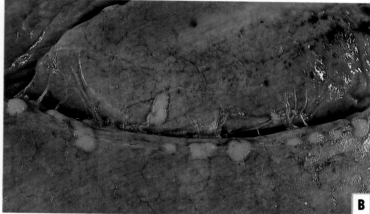

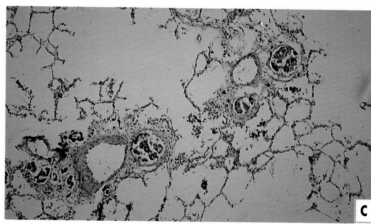

Figure 12.26 Pulmonary lymphangitic metastases. Two years after undergoing a left modified radical mastectomy, a 59-year-old patient developed shortness of breath. (A) Her chest film shows a diffuse nodular–interstitial pattern consistent with lymphangitic metastases. (B) Macroscopically, lymphangitic pulmonary metastases (from a different patient) appear as multiple yellow lesions involving lymphatic vessels. (C) Microscopically, metastatic tumor cells can be observed filling these vessels. (From Hayes, 1991.)

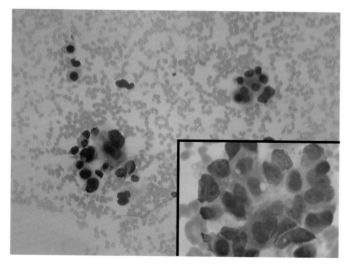

Figure 12.27 Bone marrow metastasis. Bone marrow metastases can develop with or without lytic or osteoblastic bone lesions. Anemia, leukopenia, thrombocytopenia, or various combinations of these can be the presenting clues to underlying intramedullary metastases. This low-power microscopic section of a bone marrow aspirate shows several clumps of malignant cells. At high power (inset), one clump of tumor cells demonstrates the characteristic features of metastatic carcinoma; a syncytial pattern or clumping of cells, the variable size and shape of tumor cells, and a high nucleus-to-cytoplasm ratio. The distinct, rather large nucleoli seen here may not always be present. (Courtesy of Pearl Leavitt, Administrator of Clinical Laboratories, Dana-Farber Cancer Institute, Boston, MA; from Hayes, 1991.)

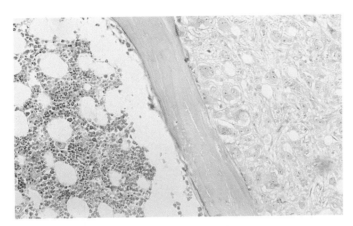

Figure 12.28 Bone marrow metastasis. A patient with known metastatic breast cancer presented with pancytopenia. Her bone marrow biopsy is shown. This figure illustrates the importance of sampling error in making the diagnosis of metastatic breast cancer. On the left side of the microscopic field, normal bone marrow was present. However, on the right side of the field, the bone marrow was replaced by metastatic adenocarcinoma consistent with a primary breast cancer.

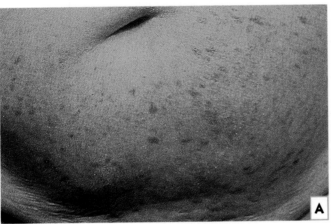

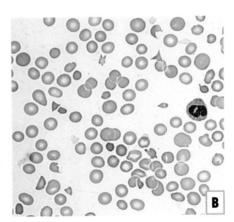

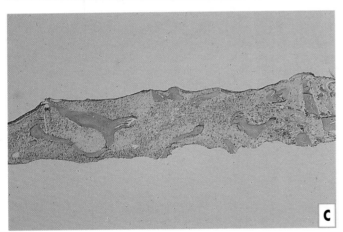

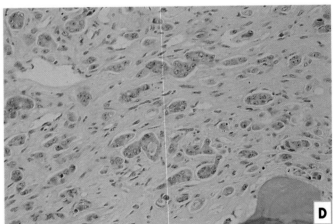

Figure 12.29 Simultaneous metastasis to multiple organs. Occasionally breast cancer metastasizes to multiple organs simultaneously, resulting in complex syndromes that are diagnostically challenging. A 63-year-old patient presented five years after a left modified radical mastectomy with complaints of fatigue, malaise, nausea, vomiting, shortness of breath, and multiple areas of bone pain. She also noted bruising, hematuria, and some blood in the stools. Physical examination revealed paleness and multiple petechiae and ecchymoses (A); she also had congestive heart failure and hepatomegaly. CT scan demonstrated diffuse hepatic metastases, and bone scan showed multiple sites of increased uptake. Her chest film was highly suggestive of lymphangitic carcinomatosis. Laboratory evaluation revealed pancytopenia, as well as hepatic and renal insufficiency. (B) Evaluation of a peripheral blood smear demonstrates a "red cell fragmentation syndrome" with many schistocytes and anisocytosis. Almost no platelets were seen, and the leukocyte count was low. She had microangiopathic hemolytic anemia. (C) Bone marrow core biopsy examination revealed almost complete replacement of hematopoietic elements with metastatic breast cancer cells, together with marked fibrosis. (D) At higher magnification, nests of tumor cells formed tubular structures within a dense fibrous stroma.

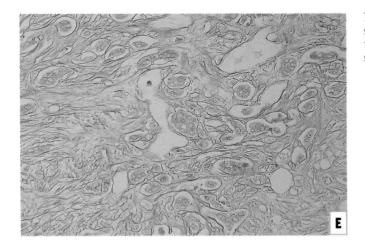

Figure 12.29, continued (E) Silver-stained section showed that nests of tumor cells were surrounded by reticulin fibers. All of her signs and symptoms could be related to widespread metastatic breast cancer. (From Hayes, 1991.)

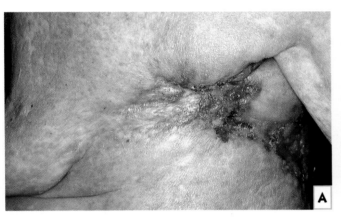

Figure 12.30 Complications of therapy. Although therapy for metastatic disease can provide palliation, the side effects of the therapy must be considered (see Chapter 9). This patient was a 74-year-old woman who presented with a far-advanced breast cancer which had led to automastectomy (A). Although tamoxifen had been previously effective in decreasing the skin ulceration and relieving her symptoms, her cancer began to progress both locally and in her bones. Within a few days of beginning hormone therapy with aminoglutethimide, she developed a widespread erythematous pruritic rash (B). Although this rash is reasonably common with the use of aminoglutethimide, it is important to remember that it frequently self-resolves. This patient's rash completely disappeared within ten days while she continued to take aminoglutethimide, and she ultimately went on to have an objective and symptomatic response.

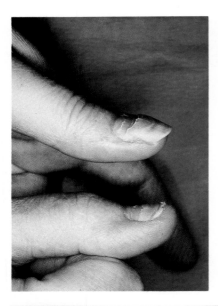

Figure 12.31 Complications of chemotherapy. Chemotherapy can also produce integumentary toxicity. This patient had metastatic breast cancer and was treated with high-dose doxorubicin. After her first course she noticed change in her fingernails. She went on to develop onycholysis and onychomadesis. Although uncommon, this is a potential complication of doxorubicin.

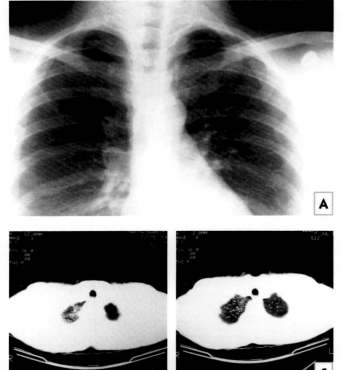

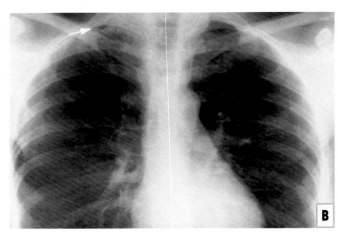

Figure 12.32 Radiation pneumonitis. Radiation therapy can be associated with local tissue damage and toxicity. This patient presented with a T_2N_3 breast cancer with supraclavicular lymphadenopathy. She was treated with lumpectomy and radiotherapy to the breast, as well as radiation therapy to the supraclavicular fossa. At that time her chest x-ray was normal (A). Two years later the patient presented with a nagging, nonproductive cough and some dyspnea on exertion. A chest x-ray (B) demonstrated a nodular right upper lobe density *(arrow)*, and a CT scan (C) confirmed the presence of these apical nodules. Bronchoscopic evaluation failed to reveal any endobronchial lesions, and a fine-needle aspiration of this area was also nondiagnostic. Over the next five years the patient did not develop any progressive symptoms or signs of malignancy. Therefore, the changes were considered to be secondary to her prior radiation, which included her right pulmonary apex.

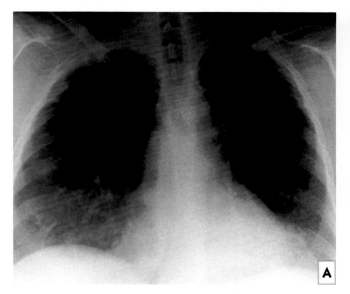

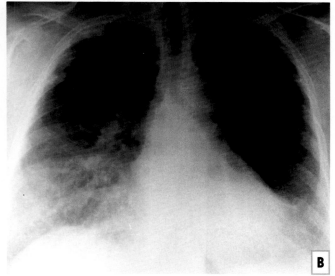

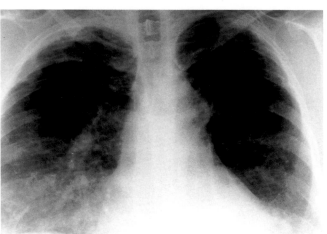

Figure 12.33 Radiation pneumonitis. This patient had a large right-sided breast cancer that was initially treated with chemotherapy, followed by radiotherapy to her right breast and chest wall. Her initial x-ray was normal (A), but at the end of her radiotherapy the patient developed a nonproductive cough and dyspnea on exertion. Chest x-ray demonstrated a right lower lobe reticulonodular infiltrate that was geometric in shape, corresponding to the radiotherapy field (B). Over the next several months, with no other therapy, the infiltrate and the patient's symptoms resolved (C).

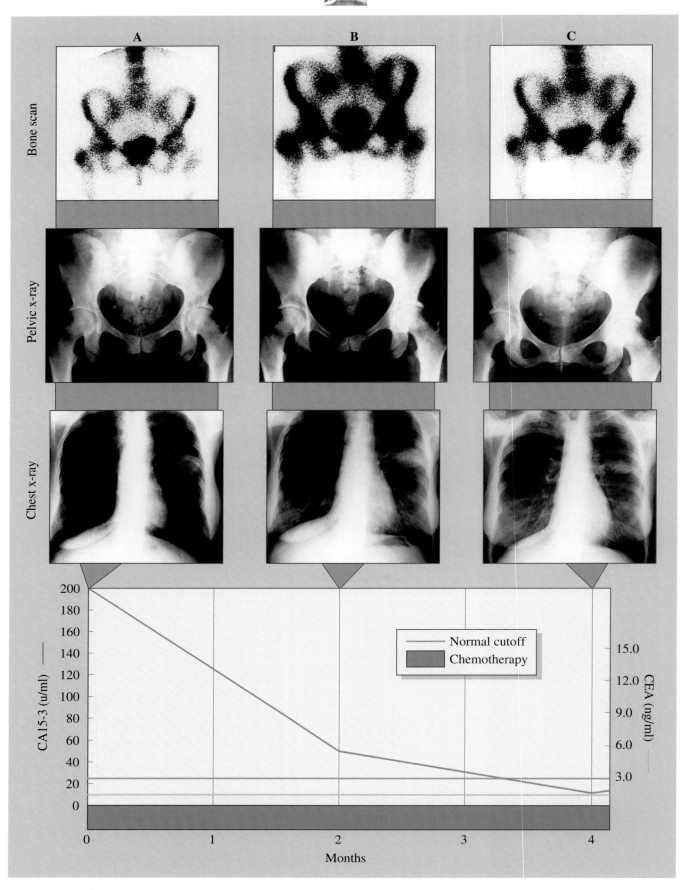

Atlas of Breast Cancer

Figure 12.34 *(at left)* Circulating tumor markers as monitors of disease course. The preceding figures have illustrated the importance of determining whether a patient is responding to therapy or whether her disease is progressing. History, physical examination, and radiographic tests can be very helpful in determining which of these is occurring. However, circulating tumor markers can also correlate with clinical disease course and can be useful in monitoring patients during therapy. In this figure, a patient with metastatic breast cancer to bone and lung (A) was initially treated with chemotherapy. Her symptoms began to resolve during the first two months of therapy, but interpretation of her physical examination, chest x-ray, and bone scans was equivocal (B). However, her CA15-3 levels decreased from an initial level of 200 U/ml to 50 U/ml. Her chemotherapy was continued, and by the fourth month of therapy she was found to be responding, as determined by history, bone scan, and chest x-ray findings (C). Of note is that the patient's CEA was never elevated and therefore in this patient was of no clinical utility.

SUGGESTED READING

American Joint Committee on Cancer. (1988) Breast. In: Beahrs OH, Henson DE, Hutter RVP, Myers MH, eds. *Manual for Staging of Cancer*, 3rd Ed. Philadelphia: JB Lippincott, 145–150.

Brinkley D, Haybittle JL, Houghton J. (1984) The Cancer Research Campaign (King's/Cambridge) trial for early breast cancer: an analysis of the radiotherapy data. *Br J Radiol* 57:309–316.

Cutler SJ. (1974) Classification of extent of disease in breast cancer. *Semin Oncol* 1:91.

Hayes DF. (1991) Breast cancer. In: Skarin A, ed. *Atlas of Diagnostic Oncology*. New York: Gower Medical Publishing.

Hayes DF, Kaplan W. (1991) Evaluation of patients following primary therapy. In: Harris J, Hellman S, Henderson I, Kinne D, (eds). *Breast Diseases*. Philadelphia, JB Lippincott, 505–525.

Henderson IC. (1991a) Chemotherapy for metastatic breast cancer. In: Harris JR, Hellman S, Henderson IC, Kinne DW, eds. *Breast Diseases*. Philadelphia: JB Lippincott, 604–665.

Henderson IC. (1991b) Endocrine therapy of metastatic breast cancer. In: Harris JR, Hellman S, Henderson IC, Kinne DW, eds. *Breast Diseases*. Philadelphia: JB Lippincott, 559–603.

Ingle JN. (1990) Principles of therapy in advanced breast cancer. *Hematol/Oncol Clin North Am* 3:743–763.

Recht A, Hayes DF. (1991) Treatment of local recurrence following mastectomy. In: Harris J, Hellman S, Henderson I, Kinne D, eds. *Breast Diseases*. Philadelphia: JB Lippincott, 527–546.

Rosen P, Groshen W, Saigo P, Kinne D, Hellman S. (1989) A long-term follow-up study of survival in stage I ($T_1N_0M_0$) and stage II ($T_1N_1M_0$) breast carcinoma. *J Clin Oncol* 7:355–366.

Stierer M, Rosen HR. (1989) Influence of early diagnosis on prognosis of recurrent breast cancer. *Cancer* 64:1128–1131.

Index

*The numbers in **bold** refer to figure numbers.*

Adenoid cystic carcinoma, 8.7, 8.8, **8.12**
Adenosis, sclerosing, **7.1**, 7.3, 7.6, **7.9**
Adjuvant systemic therapy, 11.2–11.8
Adrenalectomy, 10.8, **10.8**
   side effects of, 10.11, **10.12**
Age
   and hormone receptor content of tumors, **10.5**, 10.7
   and incidence of breast cancer, **2.1**, 2.2
Alkylating agents, 10.2, **10.3**, 10.5
Aminoglutethamide, 10.8, **10.8**
   side effects of, 10.11, **10.12**, 12.21, **12.30**
Anatomy of breast, **3.1**, 3.2
Angiosarcoma, 8.7, 8.10, **8.18**
Anthracyclines, 10.2, **10.3**, 10.5
Antimetabolites, 10.2, **10.3**, 10.5
Apocrine metaplasia, **7.1**, 7.3, 7.4, **7.4**
Arm edema, after mastectomy, 5.10, 5.11, **5.20**
Axillary dissection
   in conservative surgery, 9.6, **9.6**
   in mastectomy, 5.9–5.10, **5.16–5.17**, 5.19
Axillary lymph nodes, micrometastases to, 11.6, **11.7**, 12.2

Benign breast disorders, 7.2–7.10
   apocrine metaplasia, **7.1**, 7.3, 7.4, **7.4**
   and cancer development, **2.6**, 2.7, **7.1–7.2**, 7.3
   cysts, microscopic, **7.1**, 7.3, **7.3**, 7.4
   duct ectasia, 7.2, 7.8, **7.13**
   ductal hyperplasia, atypical, **7.1**, 7.3, 7.7, **7.10**

fat necrosis, 7.2, 7.8, **7.12**
fibroadenoma, **7.1**, 7.2, 7.3, 7.5, **7.6**
fibrocystic changes, 7.2
florid hyperplasia, **2.6**, 2.7, **7.1**, 7.3, 7.5, **7.7**
granular cell tumors, 7.2, 7.9, **7.16**
gynecomastia, 7.2, 7.10, **7.17**
hamartoma, 7.2, 7.8, **7.14**
intramammary lymph nodes, 4.9, **4.11**
lobular hyperplasia, atypical, **7.1**, 7.3, 7.7, **7.11**
mild hyperplasia, **7.1**, 7.3, 7.4, **7.5**
papilloma, intraductal, **7.1**, 7.2, 7.3, 7.6, **7.8**
radial scar, 7.2, 7.9, **7.15**
radiation effect, 7.2, 7.10, **7.18**
sclerosing adenosis, **7.1**, 7.3, 7.6, **7.9**
Biopsies, 5.2–5.4
   and analysis of hormone receptors in tumors, 6.4–6.6, **6.4–6.5**
   core needle, 5.4
      processing of, 6.2
   excisional, 5.2, **5.2**, 5.3, 5.4, **5.4**
      needle-directed, **5.2**, 5.3, 5.4, 5.5, **5.5**
      processing of, **6.1–6.3**, 6.2–6.4
   and hookwire needle localization with mammography, **4.6**, 4.6–4.7, 4.9
   incisional, 5.2, **5.2**, 5.3, 5.4, **5.4**
      processing of, 6.2
   needle aspiration, 5.2, **5.2–5.3**, 5.3
      processing of, 6.2
   and specimen radiography, **4.6**, 4.7, 4.9, 6.2, **6.3**, 6.4
   stereotactic, **5.2**, 5.3, 5.4
      fine-needle aspiration in, 4.8, **4.8**, 4.9
   techniques in, 5.2, **5.2**, 5.3
Bone marrow metastasis, 12.20, **12.28**
Bone metastases, 12.11–12.14, **12.14–12.19**
   fractures in, 12.4, 12.8, **12.9**

lytic versus blastic lesions in, 12.13, **12.17**
Brain metastases, 12.10, **12.12**

Calcifications detected in mammography, 4.5–4.8, **4.6–4.8**
   evaluation of, 4.8, 4.9, **4.9–4.10**
Cell cycle, **10.2**, 10.4
   measures of cellular turnover in, 11.6, 11.7, **11.9**
   and resistance to chemotherapy, **11.1**, 11.2
Chemotherapy, **10.1–10.3**, 10.2, 10.3–10.4, 10.5
   adjuvant, **11.2**, 11.2–11.6, **11.4–11.5**
      recommendations for, 11.5, 11.7, **11.10**
   agents in, 10.2, **10.3**, 10.5
   cell cycle stages in, **10.2**, 10.4
   combinations of agents in, 10.9, 10.10, **10.11**
   logarithmic killing of neoplastic cells in, 10.8–10.9, **10.10**
   mechanisms of action, **10.1**, 10.3
   radiotherapy with, in locally advanced cancer, 9.14, **9.23**
   resistance to, 10.8–10.9, **10.9**
      cell cycle affecting, **11.1**, 11.2
   toxicity of, 10.9–10.10, 12.10, 12.22, **12.31**
Comedo type of ductal carcinoma in situ, 8.2, 8.3, **8.3–8.4**, 8.4
Cyclophosphamide, 10.2, **10.3**, 10.5
   toxicity of, 10.9
Cystosarcoma phyllodes, 8.7, 8.10, **8.17**
Cysts, microscopic, **7.1**, 7.3, **7.3**, 7.4
Cytotoxic agents, 10.2

Development of breast cancer
   hypothetical model of, 2.7, **2.7**, 2.8
   risk with benign lesions, **2.6**, 2.7, **7.1–7.2**, 7.3